ERMANY

AUSTRIA

ALY

Florence

°Rome

Naples +
+
Ravello +
+
Bari

+
Taranto

Mediterranean Sea

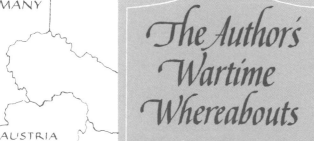

The Author's Wartime Whereabouts

+
Places visited with
American Red Cross

◉
Places visited with OSS

BETWEEN THE LINES

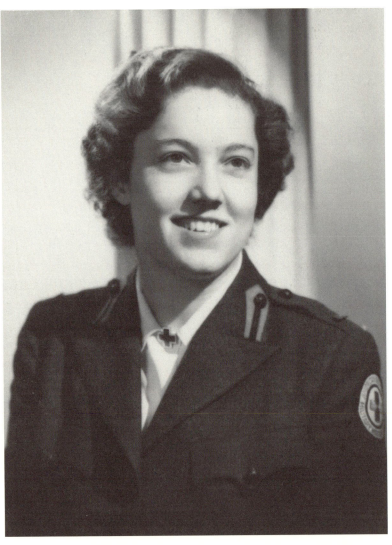

The author in American Red Cross uniform c. 1943

Between the Lines

Overseas with the Red Cross and OSS in World War II

ELIZABETH PHENIX WIESNER

Jenna
with affectionate best wishes
Lee.

Posterity Press

Posterity Press, Inc.
P.O. Box 71081
Chevy Chase, MD 20813
http//:www.posteritypress.com

Printed in the United States of America

Library of Congress Catalog Card Number: 98-065211

ISBN 1-889274-04-6

For "Dear Mother, Father, Richard and Joan"
to whom these letters were written

You trace my journeys and my resting places
And are acquainted with all my ways

Psalm 139, verse 2

Contents

Foreword

———❖———

Most of us can remember vividly where we were when critical national or international calamities occurred. When the radio announcer broke into the symphony concert on December 7, 1941, I was in a New York hospital room visiting my mother. Fifty-six years later every detail of that moment is etched in my memory.

So each of us recalls world-changing moments but not many of us have been involved in history as has Elizabeth P. Wiesner, my friend Lee. While most women stayed at home, writing V-Mail letters to unknown and mysteriously named locations around the world, Lee was writing letters home from some of those same far-away places.

Her letters were full of homely and exotic detail—how to keep clean with a cup of water in an Army helmet, descriptions of alien landscapes, flowers and people—because wherever Lee goes people flock to her, claim her as friend, confide in her, love her.

In her first book, Lee described her spiritual journey. It has been a lifelong one, but I believe it truly began when she first reached out to lonely, homesick and wounded soldiers who needed her gentle presence. She is still soothing, consoling, advising and praying for us all.

On the road that began when she accepted the American Red Cross's invitation to serve in North Africa in World War II, Lee has covered many an exciting mile. Her letters home, her diaries and her formidable memory combine in this account of her war years in Boston, Washington, North Africa and much of Europe.

For those of us of the same generation, the account revives our own memories. For those of younger generations, the book gives a memorable view of life in wartime from one young woman's perspective.

Nancy S. Montgomery
Washington, D.C.
November 1997

Preface

———◆———

Ⅰn my first book, *Pilgrim and Pioneer, A Journey with God,*[†] I traced my journey from an unchurched childhood to my ordination and some of the significant events in my life as an Episcopal priest. The time between my baptism as an adult and my marriage some ten years later, I summed up in a single paragraph, considering it interesting and sometimes exciting, but basically an irrelevant part of my "journey." However, as it referred to my assignments overseas during World War II, so many people asked me "what did you do during the war?" that I decided to try to answer the question by writing this second and frankly secular book. It is based on the many letters I wrote to my family back home, from North Africa and Italy when I was with an American Red Cross hospital unit, then from

———

† Published in 1989 by Churchman Publishing Ltd., distributed in the United States by Morehouse Publishing, and now out of print.

North Africa, Spain, England and Switzerland when I was working with the Office of Strategic Services. OSS was the United States' principal intelligence and espionage organization throughout the war, and the precursor of the Central Intelligence Agency.

For reasons of security, when my letters were written the identification of people and places was often purposely vague. In general I have let that vagueness remain. In some cases I have forgotten a person's last name; in some cases I have not been able to get in touch with them to get permission to use their names; in a few cases it didn't seem relevant or important enough to pursue the matter.

Unlike many of the now-it-can-be-told books already in print, this memoir bares no secrets. Rather it is an account of the ordinary happenings in one young American woman's daily life in the midst of the extraordinary events of a world at war. The latter from time to time touched the former, of course, even on occasion quite dramatically, as in the case of the shocking mustard gas disaster in Bari, Italy, in 1944, which is described in Chapter Three.

Books sometimes seem to have an agenda of their own, and as I gathered my material and started to write, I realized that there was a very real and significant connection between my baptism and my subsequent activities—though I did not recognize it at the time, more than fifty years ago. It never occurred to me in 1940 that my baptism was an empowerment for service to others and, therefore, I never thought of my jobs with the so-called caring professions or my volunteer work as a nurse's aide or member of the Massachusetts Women's Civilian Corps as forms of ministry. My baptism, I had felt, was a personal and almost entirely spiritual event, establishing a vertical intimate relationship between me and God. I was "marked with a cross as Christ's own forever," a child of God, "born anew of water and the Spirit," but little if anything was said about how this should influence my relationships with others. According to the 1928 Prayer Book's Offices of Instruction, I had promised "to love my neighbor as myself" but I had no sense of my neighbor as someone whom I was called to serve in any way. The Baptismal Covenant in the 1979 Book of Common Prayer now quite emphatically calls the candidate as well as the gathered community of baptized persons "to seek and serve Christ in all persons" and to "strive for justice and peace among all people and respect the dignity of every human being."

With hindsight, I can see how I was intuitively responding to this broader interpretation of the sacrament of baptism as empowering me for a form of lay ministry, especially when I went overseas with the Red Cross in early 1943. Since I didn't know consciously that that was what I was doing, I didn't call it that and my letters were just narratives of events and feelings, for the information, enjoyment and sometimes amusement of my parents and siblings.

Those letters, as I said, form the basis for this book. I have used verbatim excerpts from many of them and summarized others. I have added connecting remarks or clarifying comments not only for the information and, I hope, enjoyment of those who wanted to know more about my in-between years, but also in celebration of the 50th anniversary of the end of World War II. And, not incidentally, reflecting on these events of more than half a century ago has helped affirm my conviction that God has indeed been guiding me all my days.

Acknowledgments

———✦———

As when I wrote my first book, the College of Preachers in Washington, D. C. is again high on my list of those to whom I wish to express my deep gratitude. My six weeks there as a fellow provided quiet space, unfettered time and pleasant surroundings during the early days of sorting out my World War II letters, which form the basis of this book. The warden and president, the Reverend Dr. Erica Wood, gave me much-needed encouragement during my time there.

My longtime friends Nancy Montgomery and Diane Haddick gave generously of their time and talents during the many months it took to get the manuscript written, edited and transcribed. Lucinda Conger, another friend from the Washington Cathedral, also assisted in that process as did my brother Richard, my daughter Liz, and my good friend Greg Hancock. Many other friends and colleagues read bits and pieces of the manuscript and made comments that were most helpful; they will know who they are and will, I hope, accept this expression of my thanks.

All our work would have been left to linger unpublished

without the patient and persistent editing and guidance of my editor and publisher, Philip Kopper; the copy editor and advisor, Mary Ann Harrell; and the designer, Susan Lehmann. I am indeed grateful for all they did; the results of which the readers now hold in their hands.

Last, but far from least, I am extremely grateful to my husband Louis A. Wiesner who several times encouraged me when I was tempted to drop the whole project and who contributed his wisdom in the writing of the Introduction.

Introduction

Since most people living today were not yet born when World War II and the events recounted in this book took place, and since memories of that momentous conflict have grown fragmentary, a brief summary, even though greatly oversimplified, seems in order to put my experiences into context.

After coming to power in Germany in 1933, Adolf Hitler quickly crushed internal opposition, began his oppression of Jews and, evading or flouting the Versailles Treaty, constructed a mighty military machine. Then, through mendacious diplomacy, naked threats, manufactured public opinion, and the failure of Britain, France, and other powers to face the reality of his unbridled ambition, Hitler swallowed up Austria in March of 1938.[†] He seized the German-

† The principal sources for historical data are James Trager, *The People's Chronology* (New York: Henry Holt and Company, 1992), and J.A.S. Grenville, *A History of the World in the Twentieth Century*, (Cambridge, MA: The Belknap Press of Harvard University Press, 1994).

speaking parts (Sudetenland) of Czechoslovakia in November, and the rest of that country within six months.

World War II began in Europe on September 1, 1939, with the German military attack on Poland, to which Britain and France responded with declarations of war on September 3. After quickly dividing Poland up with the Soviet Union, Hitler's forces seemed to rest for some months; then in the spring of 1940, they overran Denmark, Norway, the Netherlands, Belgium, Luxembourg, and marched triumphantly into Paris in June. Some 338,000 British, French, and other Allied soldiers were evacuated from the beaches of Dunkirk to England, which was itself bombed by the *Luftwaffe* but stood firm. Winston Churchill and the British people were the only bulwark against what seemed to be the inevitable conquest of Western Europe by the Nazi beast. In the spring of 1941, the Germans took most of the Balkans. Then on June 22, 1941, Hitler made one of his fatal mistakes by attacking his erstwhile ally, the Soviet Union (just as Napoleon had done to Russia in June, 1812), and his forces drove deep into that vast country.

During those years, starting even before the war, the Nazis perpetrated the most vicious atrocities including the systematic persecution and genocide of the Jews and other peoples they deemed "inferior races." A total of over 14 million were thus murdered, of whom about 6 million were Jews. Nazi atrocities included massacres of civilians in retaliation for any resistance; forced labor; slaughter of "subhuman" prisoners of war in the eastern combat zones; and—most notoriously—mass deportations to the death camps, facilities especially built for the murder of thousands upon thousands of innocent prisoners, most of them the victims of the genocidal Holocaust. These war crimes became known worldwide, and in the postwar Nuremberg Trials punishment was meted out to the Nazi officials who were tried and found guilty of documented "crimes against humanity."

The war in the Pacific (which is not part of this book but was not absent from our consciousness) can be said to have begun in July 1937, when Japan resumed a campaign to conquer China, and for the first time Chiang Kai-shek resisted. Some Japanese troops committed atrocities no less horrible (though less systematic) than those of the Nazis in Europe. In September 1940, Japan, Germany and Italy signed the Tripartite Pact, which divided the world (excluding the U.S.S.R.) into spheres of influence and pledged mutual military assistance if any of the three were attacked by a power not then at war (read the United States).

The United States stayed out of both the European and Asian wars during their early years, as there was strong isolationist sentiment in this country stemming from the tragic cost and troubled aftermath of World War I. However, public opinion did support President Franklin D. Roosevelt's steadily increasing economic and military aid to Britain, much of Europe and to China, and his application of trade and financial restrictions against Japan. Diplomatic negotiations failed with Japan over its conquests and the U.S. sanctions, and on Sunday, December 7, 1941, the Japanese bombed the U.S. Pacific Fleet at Pearl Harbor, Hawaii, in a surprise attack. That "day which will live in infamy" brought a declaration of war requested by the President and overwhelmingly passed by the Congress. It was quickly followed by Hitler's declaration of war against the United States. From then on the European theater took priority in American war strategy.

The external circumstance that led to my arrival in North Africa—and the beginning of this account—was the Allied decision that caused U.S. and British forces commanded by General Dwight D. Eisenhower to land at Casablanca,

Oran, and Algiers on November 7 and 8, 1942. They quickly defeated the garrisons of the Nazi-installed Vichy French regime. Germany then occupied the Vichy territory of southern France and sent reinforcements to North Africa. However, the Germans there were defeated by May 1943, and British-U.S. forces invaded Sicily in July, pushing on to Italy later. Some of the subsequent developments are summarized later in this book.

When World War II ended in Europe on May 8, 1945, and in Asia on August 14 of that year, almost 55 million people had been killed, more than half of them civilians (including the victims of genocide). U.S. military deaths numbered 407,316, with another 670,846 wounded, according to *The World Almanac*. Most of Europe and much of Asia were devastated, and their peoples lived in appalling misery for a number of years afterward.

However, the barbarous regimes in Germany and Japan had been totally defeated and surrendered unconditionally. Led by the United States, the free world rebuilt itself and also the enemy countries. New institutions were put in place for collective security and for economic and social cooperation. One of them, NATO, successfully contained the Soviet Communist dictatorship until it collapsed in 1991. Though many international and civil wars have occurred in places around the world, including Korea, Vietnam, and the Persian Gulf, none approached the dimensions of the Second World War. Unfortunately, half a century after the end of that awful conflagration, it appears that the world community has forgotten its lessons, and is again willing to stand by while new aggressors and barbarians—in Bosnia and central Africa, for example—defy the laws of nations and commit massive crimes against humanity.

CHAPTER ONE

Here Am I, Send Me

—❖—

December 7, 1941–April 5, 1943

The attack on Pearl Harbor by the Japanese on December 7, 1941, came at the end of a year of escalating events. The most significant of these were the invasion of Yugoslavia and Greece by the Germans in early April, the landing of German paratroopers on Crete in early May, and the German attack on the Soviet Union in late June. The war itself had, of course, started in Europe in 1939, but we were not formally involved until President Roosevelt signed the declaration of war on Japan on December 8, and Hitler's declaration of war with us on December 11.

U.S. Army Air Corps planes from the carrier *Hornet* bombed Tokyo in mid-April. Gasoline, tires, shoes, sugar and meat were strictly rationed at home. Corregidor was surrendered on May 6; the Battle of Midway June 3–6 marked a decisive defeat for the Japanese; and finally on November 8, 1942, U.S. and Allied troops landed in North Africa. The presence of these troops enabled the American Red Cross to send some of its personnel directly to North Africa and to deploy others from England where they had been waiting.

I
t was late afternoon on December 19, 1942, and my annual pre-Christmas cocktail party was in full swing when the doorbell rang. One of my guests ran down the stairs to answer it and came back up

waving a yellow envelope in her hand. Telegrams in my family were never casually sent so I opened it with a certain amount of apprehension which quickly changed to excited disbelief as I read the following words:

CAN YOU COME TO RED CROSS WASHINGTON D.C. MONDAY DECEMBER 28 FOR INTERVIEW RE: FOREIGN SERVICE STOP MUST BE ABLE TO SPEAK FRENCH STOP BIRTH CERTIFICATE REQUIRED STOP IF ACCEPTED MUST BE ABLE TO REMAIN FOR TRAINING STOP WIRE COLLECT WILL REIMBURSE FOR EXPENSE OF TRIP AND FOR MAINTENANCE.

It had all begun earlier for me in Boston, as it had for so many thousands of others, with the Japanese attack on Pearl Harbor on December 7, 1941. It was, at first, a Sunday like any other Sunday: early service at the Church of the Advent, a large brunch (only we didn't call it that in those days), then a lovely long leisurely afternoon with the Sunday papers and the New York Philharmonic on the radio—Symphony No. 1 by Dmitri Shostakovich, conducted by Artur Rodzinski. Within half an hour the broadcast was interrupted with the news that an Army transport ship had been torpedoed 1,300 miles west of San Francisco. It was interrupted a second time with the news that President Roosevelt had reported the Japanese attack on Pearl Harbor. The program resumed after intermission with the Brahms Piano Concerto No. 2 played by Artur Rubinstein, which was also twice interrupted with news bulletins. Finally, transmission of the concert ended prematurely and the air was filled with updates of the attack.

As I wrote the next morning from my office (I was a medical secretary and receptionist for two ophthalmologists on Newbury Street):

Dear Mother and Father,

So it's come at last. I feel as though I was doing everything in a fog—every once in a while I peer through and am amazed that people and events seem to go on in their normal way. Being here in the office is the worst part of it, no news from 8:15 to 5:45. I sat on the stairs today to catch a few words of the President's message from the radio upstairs, but the doctor and his wife went right on eating without paying any attention to it. I am going to see at once in what way I can be useful, U.S.O. perhaps. Damn, damn damn it all. *Why* did they do it?

Finished addressing Christmas cards this morning. I feel an almost frantic compulsion to do something, anything just to quit thinking. Even the dullest job helps. But how can one put Merry Christmas and Happy New Year on them now?

It was mostly those dull jobs that kept me occupied after Japan shocked the United States out of isolationism with the sneak attack on Pearl Harbor on December 7, which President Roosevelt described the next day as "a date which will live in infamy" when he asked Congress for a declaration of war. Although the U.S. had been more than a little involved in helping Britain fight Nazi Germany, the majority of Americans still wanted to stay out of the war. As a journalist summed up fifty years later, "Japan changed all that."

I continued to work as a medical secretary although I changed jobs, leaving the ophthalmologists for an allergist. I also created a bit of personal drama by breaking my wrist in January when I fell on an icy step with my arms full of groceries, and by having a grumbling appendix out in March, thinking that if I ever did go overseas it was best to have it taken care of ahead of time. And as a Red Cross nurse's aide as well as a member of the Massachusetts Women's Civilian Defense Corps, I was called in to the Massachusetts General Hospital to help with some of the living victims of the Coconut Grove nightclub fire in which more than 400 people perished. It happened November 28, 1942, the day after the Thanksgiving Day football game and was called the holiday holocaust; some of the techniques perfected in treating these burn patients, one of whom was Charles "Buck" Jones, a popular cowboy film star, became standard procedures later.

During the previous spring and summer, I had become increasingly eager to offer my services, increasingly impatient with my dull office work and volunteer activities, and feeling a deep personal need to be of some use somewhere in some capacity, preferably overseas. "Here am I, send me"[†] became my theme as "the winds of war" (in Herman Wouk's wonderful phrase) blew ever more vigorously. Letters listing my qualifications and offering my services as a civilian secretary and/or nurse's aide to several hospitals and Red Cross offices were answered courteously, but in the negative.

In June the National Red Cross had actually sent me an application which I duly submitted, but without any real hope of acceptance. I had included an indirect reference to a knowledge of French, having had it in school since the first grade. It was that which led almost six months later to the telegram which quite literally changed my life. At last I, too, might have a chance to do something worthwhile and useful. At last someone had responded to my repeated plea, "Here am I, send me."

I suppose the party continued to run its course. I suppose I telephoned my parents in New York, and obviously I sent a telegram of acceptance to the Red Cross, but I have no recollection of anything that happened during the ten days before I went to Washington. Where did I spend Christmas? Who closed my apartment and stored my furniture? The only records I have of my activities between the arrival of that telegram and the first letter I wrote from North Africa are a few letters from Washington to my parents,

† The phrase is from Isaiah 6:8.

mostly about errands that needed to be done (by my mother) and financial matters that needed to be cleared up (by my father).

Having been accepted after my interview on December 28, I was billeted with a number of others at the Hotel Annapolis and my brief period of training began. My letters home dealt mostly with the problems of finding and buying a year's supply of everything I might need, including soap and toothpaste, and complicated by the fact I had no idea where I was going or when! Being in class until late afternoon limited my shopping so my requests to my mother were numerous, frequent and detailed. Needless to say she was a wonderful help. When we were issued our basic uniforms, being at that point a perfect size 14, I was one of the first to blossom out in "full fig." I discovered that the guards at the White House gates mistook me for a military officer of some sort and would salute smartly as I walked past, which I did quite often and quite unnecessarily.

I was given ten days of embarkation leave with my parents in New York during which time I finished my shopping, saw many friends and relatives and, a bit to my surprise, became engaged to a young doctor from Massachusetts General Hospital in Boston whom I had met the previous year when I was a patient there. Not a very sensible thing to do with at least a year's separation ahead of us, but the heart knows no reasons and has its own seasons and it was somehow comforting to have this additional tie to home. (And, of course, we were very much in love.)

The last night in the United States was spent by our Red Cross unit at the Hotel St. George on Brooklyn Heights, just a few blocks from where I had lived as a teenager and where I had attended Packer Collegiate Institute. Our group left the hotel in big Army trucks, "quietly and at night," as I wrote in my journal. Once down at the docks we marched in formation up the slippery gangplank, each of us laden down with gas mask, canteen, pistol belt, musette bag (a heavy canvas and leather bag with carrying straps) and suitcase, and the pockets of our Army issue greatcoats stuffed with all the last-minute odds and ends we hadn't been able to fit in elsewhere. Our ship was the USAT (United States Army Transport) *Acadia,* formerly of the Fall River Line, that used to ply between Fall River, Massachusetts and New York. It was being used as a troopship on the way over to Africa and a hospital ship on the way back. As I remember, this was its maiden ocean voyage; that fact, plus its very small size, only added to our apprehension about the safety of a midwinter crossing of the submarine-infested Atlantic to an unknown destination.

We "upped anchor," my journal goes on to say, "early in the morning of February 8, 1943." No one was allowed on deck until after we had passed Ambrose Light so I missed the familiar sights of the harbor and a last glimpse of land. I was billeted in an inside room with five other Red Cross workers: Lillian McLeod, Marie Louise Morrison, Jo McNamara, Blanche Novak and Kathleen Perkins. Blanche later joined the Foreign Service but I've been unable to discover her present whereabouts, nor have I been able to find the other four through Red Cross records.

The doctors and nurses who were part of the ship's hospital component had little with which to occupy themselves on the way over. So when I bumped my head coming up from the troop mess hall where I had been passing out ditty bags containing toiletries and cigarettes they all "came hurrying around at a run" as A. A. Milne phrased it in a poem. I was promptly put to bed in a hospital ward with special nurses on eight-hour shifts and submitted to various tests to see if perhaps I had a skull fracture or maybe a subdural hematoma. Back rubs, bed baths, special meals, fruit juice on demand—it was a welcome diversion for all of us for several days. What a comedown later when, after I had been discharged to my crowded quarters (having been diagnosed most disappointingly from their standpoint as having merely a mild concussion), I developed unmistakable symptoms of jaundice. It probably resulted from the yellow fever shots we all received in Washington, according to Lt. Walter Casale, one of the doctors whom I remember with special gratitude. Being on a special lowfat, very unappetizing diet, I had to eat my meals in the hospital office which was much nicer and more fun than the crowded officers' mess. I was allowed to help myself from a special supply of fruit juices and canned peaches that was kept in the fridge just for me. I did some typing of news bulletins for Sgt. Maj. Ray Beauvais and, all in all, it was a pleasantly uneventful trip, even though the lovely moonlit nights caused a bit of concern for fear of U-boat attack.

Landfall toward midnight on February 19; I wrote in my journal:

Dark and very mysterious. Africa rose out of the water and mist. Made me feel very queer. Saw the coast of Spain but the decks were cleared about 3 AM so I missed Gibraltar. We were fired on from shore once. I wasn't really scared, just cold in my stomach.

On February 21 I wrote, "Landed in Oran this morning! Beautiful harbor. Taken to town in trucks. Billeted in an old maternity hospital. Gave a dance this afternoon at the Service Club." Three days later I wrote my first letter home headed "Somewhere in North Africa." I commented on how dirty and dusty or muddy Oran was and how quickly my French was coming back, especially practical words like *papier hygiénique* (not immediately necessary as Walter Casale gave me nine rolls from the ship).

I was assigned at first to one of the enlisted men's clubs to work with Helene Finan and Elaine Jackson; our hours were from 9 A.M. to 10 P.M. or even midnight. I had been appointed PX (Post Exchange) officer, which meant going to the warehouse and shopping in quantities and running a "clinic" one evening for several enlisted men with cuts of varying severity, a merchant seaman with pulmonary tuberculosis whom I finally got admitted to the hospital, and a drunk sailor who had stumbled on glass. My comment on it all was "life is never dull" and it was a "really good evening!"

A letter to my family written March 4 went into more detail:

They have billeted us in what used to be a maternity hospital! What a lot of teasing we get because of that. But it will really be quite a comfortable place when they get it all fixed up. Right now there is no hot water, no baths, one W.C. that works spasmodically, the beds (as a good maternity bed should) all hump up in the middle like a camel, and until last night we had no sheets or pillowcases.

The flowers here (I have a big bunch on my desk which made me think of it) are lovely. Violets are sold on the street, a big bunch for twenty francs. Then a French woman gave me some paper-white narcissus the other day, just stopped and pressed them into my hands without saying a word.

I got interrupted, by what I do not remember now. It might have been when I rushed out to do a little first aid for a soldier who fell down 40 stone steps and got a lovely cut over his eye, or it might have been to drive out in a two-and-a-half-ton truck about 30 miles to find some people, only to discover that they had left, and then my driver seemed to be acting rather peculiarly so a lieutenant drove me home in a jeep with the truck following me and we got lost and didn't get home until very late and everybody was just about to send out a searching party or something.

That brings me to my newest news—that I am being

transferred from the club out into a hospital unit! I am so pleased—I'm going to be living in a tent and eating out of my mess kit all the time and washing in my helmet and probably wearing boots and coveralls and I'm so pleased and excited! Aren't I silly to be glad to leave a bed and sheets for a camp cot and bedroll?

I moved out the next day to join the 26th General Hospital, which was composed of medical and dental staff from the University of Minnesota Medical School. My enthusiasm with my assignment is obvious from the way I wrote my family some days later:

Dear Mother, Father, Richard and Joan—

My, how fast things change here. Tonight, six o'clock, having just finished chow, I am sitting on the ground in front of my tent with the late afternoon sun warm on my back as I write you. My typewriter is balanced in front of me on a non-stable rock, so any mistakes I make you may blame on that. I really do feel like a newspaper correspondent now. And you should see what I have on! A nice little hat that is called a fatigue hat over here but in the States all the girls are wearing them (maybe you have one, Joan) and they are called jeep hats. Then I have on a nice warm O.D. [olive drab] men's shirt with a field jacket over that, warm O.D. men's pants (I can never remember to keep the fly buttoned, it's an awful nuisance, really!), wool socks and heavy men's shoes that remind me of my favorite ski boots. All G.I. [government issue] stuff and very comfortable. To that tomorrow I will add coveralls and leggings! You know how I love to wear slacks anyway, so I am simply in heaven. And all the lovely uniforms that they issued me in Washington are in my blanket roll to make it more comfortable to sleep on! And all my shoes, including those lovely white ones we bought, Mother, are in the bottom of my barracks bag (which item now replaces my footlocker, which I am checking in one of the Red Cross clubs with my civilian clothes until that far-away day when I either go back to the USA or take a vacation and go to Cairo or something).

Numerous activities are going on around me, girls writing letters, some knitting; laundry is suspended from the tent ropes and some of the girls washed their hair this afternoon, using their helmets for that purpose as well as for sponge baths, washing clothes and the more usual use of the helmet of protecting the head! To my left are a few tents, then a slope down to the road and more tents up the side of the little hill beyond. And in front of me a green and fertile valley with gentle hills beyond, all checker-boarded with green fields, brown earth and cut-down vineyards. And in the far distance on the other side some mountains that look strange and artificial with their flat tops. The countryside as I drove out here the other day is filled with an incredible number of all variety of flowers—it looks somewhat like California in the springtime with the poppies and lupine, only here I don't know the names of the flowers. I will try to get some and really press them and send them to you. We can use them for slides when I give my lectures on North Africa after the War.

After the dampness and dankness of town, even though I loved it with its interesting people and color and picturesqueness, this place is heaven. I've been out in the sun almost all day and it's wonderful. So far we have no work to do, and this is just a staging area. And after the long hours I had in the club, from nine in the morning until ten or later at night with no time to oneself (I had about decided that I would join a convent when I got back, just to get away from men) it is elegant to be able to sit and look at a hill or lie on one's cot or stand and talk to a friend. I'm hoping that all this sun will bake away the rest of my cold. Now the danger is over, I can tell you that I was exposed to mumps on the way over! I was terribly afraid that I would get them, having jaundice at the time I thought would probably lower my resistance to infection. But the three weeks period from the day I was exposed is over and I haven't got them. I was very glad. I did not come to Africa to have the mumps; concussion and jaundice are plenty for the time being.

My new outfit is the 26th General Hospital, so I am no longer a linguistic secretary but a hospital secretary which of course makes me very happy. It seems like a very grand group and I'm terribly pleased. I am half a recreation worker and half a secretary as I am taking the place of two girls who didn't enjoy either the work or the living conditions and had asked to be transferred into Oran. I requested my transfer but I was very much surprised when I got it. The Red Cross is too much like the Army for one to expect things like that.

We live in big ward tents with 18 girls to a tent. We sleep on cots with straw mattresses and five blankets in good old envelope style, just as we used to do on camping trips except we don't have big safety pins for the sides. I have put my lovely blanket [a beautiful soft red plaid cashmere from Abercrombie & Fitch which I still have and treasure] on the very inside and shall use it tonight for the first time. I can hardly wait to go to bed. Oh, I forgot, the bed roll goes on the straw mattress before the blankets. Inside the roll we keep all our soft clothes. One's underwear etc. goes in bed with one to keep it warm and dry for the morning as it is quite damp at night. But somehow dampness in a tent is much nicer than dampness in a stone building with stone floors. Everything is really quite cozy—we have a small garden out in front of the tent and some tin cans serve as vases inside. Some of the girls in another tent have collected about a dozen turtles which they have painted white with their names on in red nail polish! And there are several dogs and a goat and a young lamb.

Our meals we eat out of our mess kits. The two plates go in one hand, the cup in another and the utensils (you soon learn to eat everything with the spoon to save washing and changing from one utensil to another) go in a pocket of the field jacket. You stand in a long line (as for everything) and walk past the steaming pots of food. It is ladled out as you go by, everything from hash (or Spam as it may be) to jam and coffee and milk and sugar. Then you go on up the hill to a long wooden trestle that is chest high at which you stand while you eat (rain or shine!), then another line past the garbage pail where you dump what you haven't eaten, to the three big kettles over the fire in which you wash rinse and rinse again your dishes. And, silly me, I love it all. This, to my foolish mind, is much more fun than what I was doing and when work begins, it will be much more valuable work. I am not belittling the work of the clubs, because I think it is very important, but hospital work is even more so. And you know how I like hospitals anyway. The kids on the boat said I got sick on purpose just so that I could be around in a medical environment.

The sun is just setting and it is rapidly getting cold, so I will have to stop. An Arab with two donkeys is just coming over the hill—a little earlier there was a whole family, including baby in mother's arms, all very colorfully dressed. I cannot tell you how happy and content I am. Only at mail time when no letters come for me, do I feel homesick. I expect they will come in a big batch one of these days.

My love to you all, Father, Mother, Richard and Joan. I do miss you—but I wouldn't miss this for anything!

On Sunday, March 15, I wrote:

What a perfectly beautiful day this has been. Yesterday was kind of cold and rainy, clearing up in the early evening with a lovely sunset, and today has been just like spring. We get up about seven, with breakfast at seven-thirty, and while we are standing there eating, the sun comes up over the hill. Even if the food wasn't good, which it is, it would be worth getting up for, just to see the sun come up. And anyway, we go to bed so early that by seven I am ready to get up. There is just a little hesitation because the bed is so nice and warm, and the tent at that hour is quite dark and cold and damp. Then we came back to the tent and fixed it up for tent inspection (I feel as if I were at summer camp and writing home about the daily routine!). I went to the Catholic church services at nine o'clock with one of the girls, came back and puttered around for an hour, making a couple of bags to put things in (like Winnie the Pooh and his jar of honey), then to the Protestant services which were held up on the side of a hill. We had a small organ, a P.A. system (which did not work very well), a quartet of really very nice voices and a very good sermon by our chaplain. The sun by that time was nice and warm and the view was lovely and all in all it was one of the nicest church services I have ever been to. I was surprised, too, at how many people turned out for it.

By the time church was over it was almost time for lunch. Oh, I might as well give you our menus too. For breakfast we had an orange, (some mornings it is tomato juice or grapefruit juice, non-sweetened too) and they give it to us first and one has to drink it rather rapidly while moving down the chow line having the rest of the food put in one's mess kit. It is quite an art to drink, walk, and not tip the mess kit all at the same time. We have cornflakes or oatmeal or something similar with sugar and canned milk, French toast with bacon (sometimes it is pancakes or scrambled eggs or sort of an omelette with sausage in it) and coffee. For supper tonight there was Spam. (While I was in town we had that three times a day, fixed in every imaginable fashion and some that were not imaginable. I never did like the stuff anyway and now I am becoming quite allergic to it. It seems to be almost the staple food of the Army and imagine what one poor fellow felt when he got a package from home and opened it with great excitement to find it contained nothing but Spam!) Anyway, the Spam tonight was done the only way I like, rolled in a batter and fried. Then we had fresh peas(!) and canned corn and mashed potatoes and bread and peanut butter and canned peaches and cocoa. So you can see that we are not either underfed or badly fed. In fact I would guess that I was probably gaining a bit of weight, which I expect I will lose as soon as we start working.

13

Well, to get off the subject of food, after lunch about ten of us from my tent packed a couple of baskets with books and knitting and sandwiches we had saved from lunch and oranges which we bought from some Arabs the other day, and set off for a walk. We walked a couple of miles up a winding muddy road to the top of a hill and bivouacked there for the afternoon, wandering in a radius of a half mile or so, picking flowers and looking at the view and just soaking in the sunshine. As I have said before, the flowers are incredible. We named them according to the flowers we are familiar with and which they most resemble. So we say that we picked violets and buttercups and daisies and crocuses and calendulas and orchids. The little orchids are darling, some brown and furry, looking so much like a small bumblebee that at first we were afraid to pick them. We are going to press some of the flowers and send them out for Easter cards, so if they come through, you will see them.

Just below us where we were sitting on the side of the hill, was a neatly cultivated field and after an hour or so an Arab rode up on his tiny burro. He was sitting in a very dignified manner sidesaddle on a homemade saddle of burlap and wood, with his robes arranged around him and his white headdress. He nodded at us and greeted us in the patois French they speak and looked very pleased when I answered him. Then he let his burro wander off to graze while he sat down to cut some brush. A little later a man and a woman came along while we were picking flowers and another man walked over and asked if we had any cigarettes. My negative reply almost pleased him as I answered him in French. And the children one meets almost fall over in astonishment when I speak to them. They will make some remark about the Croix Rouge, thinking I cannot understand them, and then I speak to them, just for the fun of watching their faces.

What I started to say about the burro was that they are so small and the people look so big, that it would look better if the man carried the burro than the other way around.

My balancing system is not as good tonight, and then there are a couple of planes stunting over our heads. The pilots are friends of some of the girls and are trying to amuse us, I guess, by seeing how close to the top of the tents they can come. The planes are big and the pilots are skillful, so there is not much more than a few feet clearance—I have a tendency to duck each time.

We stayed out all afternoon and came home just in time for supper. Hungry, hot, sunburned and a little footsore. And feeling very definitely that it was a funny way to spend a Sunday afternoon in Africa in the middle of a war. At times here it seems as if we were even farther away from everything here than we were before.

My love to you all—Elizabeth.

On March 18 we were told that our hospital was to move to a site just north of the city of Constantine and fairly close to the front lines in order to receive casualties from the Tunisian campaign. Even the prospect of the long, crowded and certainly uncomfortable train ride didn't dampen my excitement. What did dampen it was the discovery, the day before we were to leave, that I had measles (for the second time yet!) and was sent bag and baggage into the officers' ward of the hospital in Oran. A very miserable ten days went by before I was allowed out of isolation and I spent my last night in the hospital taking care of a woman in the bed next to mine who was two months pregnant and miscarrying. The hospital was so short-staffed that I was even asked to take her pulse and monitor her respiration during the night.

Tom Irving, one of the Red Cross regional directors, and I flew to Algiers on Saturday, April 3, (my first-ever plane trip!) and on Monday, April 5, I drove to Constantine with Al Fincke, the Red Cross field director for our district. A beautiful drive with incredible scenery all the way. We stopped in a little village and had a drink at a café whose proprietor had once had a bar on 113th Street in New York! In Constantine I was met by Mary Mock, the assistant field director in charge of the hospital Red Cross unit, and taken out to where our hospital was being most efficiently set up. It was still in tents but with electricity and cement floors in the wards and Nissen huts [corrugated iron prefabs with half-round arching roofs] for special installations such as the operating theaters. The officers, with whom we were unofficially grouped, were assigned two to a wall tent which seemed quite luxuriously private and spacious, at least at first. It was wonderful to be "home" with my outfit again.

CHAPTER TWO

African Adventure

***

April 25–November 24, 1943

War was a way of life by 1943, on the home front as well as overseas. In contrast to the frustration of ration stamps and the short supply of many necessities, war bond rallies and scrap metal drives became popular events. In addition, there was a dramatic social impact resulting from the employment of women in the various war-related industries.

Allied forces were taking the initiative on both fronts. Some of the significant events in this turning of the tide were the bombing of Germany, the offensives in the Pacific, and the Allied landings in Sicily and Italy which had followed the departure in May of all Axis troops from North Africa. The 26th General Hospital, to which I had been assigned and which had been handling casualties from the final phase of the North African campaign, was moved to Bari in southern Italy in November.

According to a pre-war *Guide Bleu*, the Algerian city of Constantine is located 80 kilometers from the sea. Its site is a most unusual one, on a rock plateau in the shape of an island surrounded by high slopes. . . . The Rummel River encased in a deep ravine runs along two sides, another deep ravine makes the third side also inaccessible. The city is accessible only on the fourth side by a narrow isthmus and by several bridges one of which was built in Roman times and another more recent high suspension bridge. There is also the long curved viaduct of Sidi Rached. Altogether the cliff of Constantine forms a natural fortress of a strange and startling appearance.

A contributor to our hospital's official history[†] wrote:

Constantine was a city never to forget! An Arab writer has said "Like a bracelet which surrounds the arm, a river, roaring at the bottom of an inaccessible ravine, encloses that city like the mountain crags protect the raven's nest."

When we visited Constantine we came to it by the *Route de la Corniche*, a picturesque highway which approached the city by a winding course up the hills from the valleys. The road was lined with eucalyptus trees as it climbed the hills. Reaching *Djebel Sidi M'Cid*, across the ravine from the city it cut into the sheer rocky wall of the canyon; at times it passed through short tunnels, and then was built out to overhang the gorge.

A trip through the gorge itself made an interesting expedition. Entering the ravine beneath the *Pont de Sidi Rached*, we followed a pathway which traversed the length of the gorge. We followed a narrow catwalk along the steep cliffs and into the shadows of a series of natural bridges or travertine arches which covered the Rummel, (causing the ancient Berbers to name it the *Souf Djimar* or Hidden River). There were remains of Roman structures and a number of springs and finally the cascades of *Sidi M'Cid* where the waters of the Rummel leaped into the valley.

The streets of Constantine were always interesting, crowded with a polyglot population in strange garments. There were brown-eyed Arabs and blue-eyed Berbers in ori-

---

† George S. Bergh, MD, and Reuben F. Erickson, eds., *A History of the 26th General Hospital* (Minneapolis, Bureau of Engraving, undated) 91-94.

ental garb, Frenchmen in western dress, veiled women in sheet-like robes, gendarmes and soldiers: American, British, French and French Colonials (Zouaves, Tirailleurs, Algerians, Spahis and Senegalese). French troops wore American uniforms but many of the colonists still wore their picturesque costumes.

As we walked the streets of Constantine we thought what an impregnable fortress it must have been before the days of modern warfare. Men had lived there since pre-historic days. Known as Cirta then, it was the capital of Numidia. Later it was the capital of a Roman colony. It had always been a rich market city, situated between the nomads of the south and the agricultural tribes of the north. During the periods of strife of the third century it declined, but early in the fourth century it was rebuilt by Constantine the Great, from whom it takes its present name. Countless invaders have engulfed North Africa but Constantine has remained always a great city. Berbers, Romans, Carthaginians, Vandals, Arabs, Turks and now the French, all have left their imprint on it. In spite of wars, invasions and sieges, the city on the rock survives and grows greater.

We in the Red Cross unit of the 26th General Hospital grew to know this "city on the rock" very well indeed. As the proud "owners" of a real automobile, a veteran Plymouth of uncertain age and checkered career, one or the other of us made frequent trips to town, to do errands in the native quarter which was off limits to military personnel, to see friends, to visit the Red Cross Club or the field director's office, to attend church in a real building rather than a tent or on an open hillside, or just to explore various points of interest and the tiny shops.

For example, I was often asked to act as an interpreter on various shopping expeditions and as a result became quite friendly with many of the local merchants. As I wrote in a letter on April 16, when they saw me coming they would dust off their best chair (usually their only chair!), shake hands with me vigorously (a custom on coming and going and sometimes in between and something not to be neglected), do everything but kiss me on both cheeks, and proceed to make me acquainted with every detail of their business and family life. And they expect me to perform miracles.

One pottery-jar/basket/stuffed-date vendor wanted me to obtain cellophane from the United States for him. The only refusal he could understand was that it was *bloqué* which I decided meant rationed. Almost everything here seemed to be *bloqué, fini* or *ne marche pas*. One got quite frustrated at first then one developed a philosophical attitude of *n'importe* or *demain*. On one occasion I had to take 32 watches to a jeweler to be repaired; it took a solid two hours to turn them over to him! The French didn't like to rush business so we had to sit down and have a cigarette, each watch had to be discussed individually and at length, he had to tell me what he thought about the Arabs ("*les sauvages*") and to give me the latest news about his family, and finally prices were discussed.

Although initially I found my school French somewhat inadequate, I was able to enlarge my practical vocabulary on subsequent trips as I tried to fulfill numerous commissions such as going to cabinetmakers for bureaus and bookcases, to dealers in copper and tin ware, to rug merchants for grass mats for our tents, French books for our library and the post office for money orders. Everywhere my negotiations were somewhat handicapped by the need to maintain an air of quiet dignity while surrounded by numerous small native children trying to give me a shoeshine or pulling at my sleeve as they begged for candy or "chew gum." And my progress from shop to shop was hindered by all the dis-

tracting scenes around me: a lovely mosque, a quiet courtyard, donkeys clattering down the precipitous street or the
astonishing sight of an Arab in turban and burnoose working away on a Singer sewing machine!

On April 25 I wrote home:

Easter Sunday in North Africa! It really does seem incredible. Today is hot and breathless, and I am down in the office
tent all dressed up in my nice gray seersucker tropical suit! As
I am now a hospital secretary and as no hospital uniforms were
issued to me in Washington, I shall have to wear these suits
as my so-called indoor hospital dress. No real work as yet, I
mean no conventional secretarial work, but we expect the Big
Day to come soon and we have all been very busy trying to
get things in shape. I expect my duties will be much more
than that of a Red Cross secretary. Until we get one more girl,
a recreational worker, I am half that, and two days ago I was
loaned out all afternoon on "detached service" to the nursing
staff to help them get beds made up and everything set up in
the wards. My nurse's aide training came in very handy and
they have threatened to call on me again if they need help.

And I hope they do. Then all the doctors shouted with
glee when they learned that I was a medical secretary and it
is quite possible that I may be called on to take some medical
dictation. That might be fun too. My prowess as a carpenter
and painter is shown by some of the furniture here in the
office tent, which is also the patients' reading room and will
be the recreation room until the other tent gets fixed up.
With what scraps of discarded lumber we could scavenge
from around the camp area we built a cabinet in which to
put office supplies, book cases for our library, little stools, and
even a Ping-Pong table! Then we had to pull all sorts of
wires and acquire some paint in town to paint them with.
The result is a little startling but at least it is colorful. The
Ping-Pong table is green with a red edge, my cabinet is a
pale green, some of the tables are blue, the bookcases are red

with buff linings! And, as I always did as a child, I got paint on my shoes, all over my coveralls, splashed my arms with it and even got some pale green in my hair! But I had an awful lot of fun, and thought to myself, "Where else could a medical secretary sit out in the sun (mostly standing on my head, I mean), dressed in coveralls and happily daub paint all over herself and the furniture?" And that is why you sent me to Bryant and Stratton [secretarial school], Father!

That last paragraph started out with the weather; today may be sunny but for the last two days we have had the most unbelievable rain you ever saw. Just down in sheets it came. At night the sound on the roof of my tent was rather cozy but during the day it made life difficult if amusing. The earth here is really clay and the consistency that it gets when mixed with a good rain is extraordinary. The mud comes up almost over our high shoes, it is so slippery that going uphill one has to go sideways, and if you stand still for a few moments you get almost rooted and have to draw your foot out with a loud sucking sound. Everything and everybody gets covered with the stuff; you have to take your shoes off every time you go into your tent, so you learn to leave near the tent flap those things you need during the day so that you can reach them without going in, and when you go "home" you make sure that you don't have to go out again until morning. When you go calling, you back into your hostess' tent, sit on the floor and leave your feet sticking out in the rain. But it really is funny and I get the giggles watching people slip and slide down the chow line and wish that I had a movie camera so that I could see myself. Yesterday when I went home to lunch I found that we did not have a ditch around our tent and the accumulated rain from up the hill was running merrily through it. So as soon as we had eaten I grabbed a shovel, with a very long and unwieldy handle, and spent my siesta digging a big and lovely ditch. It was very satisfactory, digging out the reddish clay and gradually diverting the water from our tent to more desirable channels.

I ended one letter by trying to reassure my family that I wasn't
pining away from homesickness or anything. I doubt if I have ever done as much satisfying work before in my whole life and under such vital and interesting and exciting conditions. I am very happy, even if that does sound like a funny thing to say considering that there is a bloody and brutal war waging not too far away and much of what I do is a direct result of that.

In a letter written on May 2, the day before my 26th birthday, I described my work at the hospital in more detail. As I was writing,

a new French patient came up and wanted to know, in French of course, if we had a violin here so that he could play . . . he is, another Frenchman said, the French Charlie Chaplin. Buff, our recreation worker, lured him off into a corner to play "*les dames chinoises*" (Chinese Checkers to you), and they are having a lovely time. Buff's French is somewhat limited but that doesn't stop her at all. On the floor in front of me two Arab patients are sitting cross-legged playing chess. They are in their pajamas and bathrobes, one of them has his cap on and both of them have taken off their shoes, the better to concentrate I guess, and the effect is really most droll. The grass rug, the swarthy Arabs, the purple bathrobes and the bare toes sticking up by their knees!

I had thought that becoming a secretary in a hospital would relieve me of many of my interpreting duties but it isn't so. We have a great many French patients, some of them really French, but a lot of them Arabs or something who speak a very bastard French which is almost impossible to understand. Most of the doctors speak no French at all and very few of the nurses, so they call on me or Mary Mock to help out, particularly when they are admitting patients. Poor Mary got stuck the other night with a patient who was quite sick and the doctor wanted to know how many times he had vomited or had urinated the day before. Mary's French was learned in a convent and she had no idea how to say that so they had to try to get the meaning across by noises and gestures. It must have been hilarious. But I'm glad it wasn't me!

There was seldom a dull moment from reveille at 5:30 A.M.—I never responded until 7 when I went to breakfast dressed in coveralls over my pajamas—until 8 or 8:30 P.M. It was even later on the twice-weekly movie nights on the hillside above our tents, as we had to help with wheelchairs, see that the ambulatory patients got seats and find blankets for them if it grew chilly as it often did after nightfall. In one letter I wrote:

I think for the first time I have found a job that will hold my interest and leave me without too much excess energy by the end of the day. There is never a dull moment and my job changes from hour to hour. I am secretary/interpreter, I play Ping-Pong, checkers, rummy, I take the radio or victrola around to some of the wards where there are bed patients and give them a "concert," I write letters for those who cannot write their own. I am in charge of the library half the time, I give out razors, toothbrushes, cigarettes and such to those who need them . . . so it goes. And I love it!

Later in the month I was even busier as three days a week of my time were "traded for one Plymouth car (1937) and an urgent call for a recreation worker. I figured that that made me worth a little more than two cars and two recreation workers."

Every other day I commuted to town in a jeep or the mail car and worked a very full and long day in the regional Red Cross office with Al Fincke, with whom I had driven up from Algiers in April. Then, on the four days I was at the hospital, I had to do much of the work that had usually taken all week and be a part-time recreation worker as well!

During the final drive of the Tunisian campaign most of our patients were infantrymen who told gruesome tales of treacherous mines and boobytraps, of lying helpless for hours before litter bearers had been able to bring them back to the aid station from which they were moved through an evacuation hospital before reaching us. The British took Tunis on May 7 and mass surrenders of German and Italian troops continued until May 13; on the following day the communiqué from Allied Forces Headquarters stated, "No Axis forces remain in North Africa who are not prisoners in our hands."

In my journal I wrote on May 7:

Tunis and Bizerte fell today. I'll never forget the quiet tent, the funny light from the unshaded bulbs, the tense faces of the 50 or so men, most of them in their purple bath robes, with bandaged hands, eye shields, crutches, casts on arms and so forth as we all silently listened to the 7 o'clock news. When the announcement came, there was a loud sigh of relaxation before the excited comments and cheers began. A very dramatic and not to be forgotten moment.

On May 18 we began admitting groups of German and Italian prisoners of war who needed medical or surgical treatment of some sort. It was distressing to realize the bitter, antagonistic and even revengeful attitude of some of our American patients. The prisoners were segregated in wards within a barbed-wire fence and were, of course, closely guarded. I wrote in my journal that they seemed very young and some were obviously very sick.

Another new and quite different experience came later in the month when after a long day working in the office in Oran I was asked if I would go out to help one of the Club-mobiles take care of some 5,000 men who were bivouacked about 40 miles out of town. My earlier feelings of superiority over the "glamour girls" soon changed to great admiration for their stamina and never- failing cheerfulness. The long letter I wrote home about this was printed in the *New York Herald Tribune* on September 19, 1943:

NORTH AFRICA—One of the most publicized of overseas Red Cross activities is the coffee and doughnuts business handled by the "glamour girls" of the Clubmobiles. Here in North Africa some of the Red Cross personnel feel that the supplies and girls were urgently needed elsewhere.

As a hospital secretary I myself felt this to be so until a few nights ago, when I was asked if I would help feed some 5,000 men bivouacked about forty miles out of town. After a hasty supper some of us piled into the Red Cross truck and drove out at sunset. We passed one big group of prisoners, Germans and Italians, heavily loaded down with packs and equipment, with only two or three guards for the whole bunch. They looked up and watched us drive past with curiosity only, no dislike or fear.

As soon as we reached the bivouac area we split up. By grapevine the news was going from hill to hill that the Red Cross was here with coffee and doughnuts. Al Fincke, Red Cross regional field supervisor, who was doing a kind of courier service in the jeep, came across some men who facetiously called out, "Where are your doughnuts?" Al answered "Right over there!" They stared incredulously until they caught a glimpse of a gray uniform skirt. Their eyes opened wider. "Real American girls—out here? Come on guys! What're we waiting for?" And they took off on the run.

After three hours of smiling and of quick responses to friendly wisecracks, of handing out two doughnuts to each guy and stirring his cup of coffee as he passed down the line, of offering V-mail forms and copies of "The Stars and Stripes," and of answering the incessant question "Where are you from?"—I was ready to take back all that I ever had said or thought about the soft job of clubmobilers.

It was not the doughnuts that mattered to the men, or the coffee. It was partly the urge for companionship, for something far removed from foxholes and canned food, that made them pass along the line two or even four times. When the doughnuts ran out and the coffee was mostly grounds, they came back and smiled at us as they went by. Of course it was fun—but it was very real work too. Not the kind of work that is measured by the number of letters written or the number of loans made, but work of the kind that is measured by intangibles. I had put in a long day at the "office" but so had the other girls, meeting bombing missions with their clubmobile, and driving to the outskirts of airfields with books, magazines and games, as well as food.

One of the things that impressed me most was the unfailing politeness and good behavior of the men. Without any exception these thousands of men, just back from the front, treated the two of us with the same teasing protectiveness they would have given a kid sister. One of them attached himself to me as a sort of bodyguard, and he was quick to frown on any boy who he thought was a little too forward in his remarks. All of them were eager to run errands for me, or to move boxes or pour milk or dish out sugar. And all of them said "Thank you!" Two British Tommies outdid all the rest by coming up in their best drawing-room manner after they had finished, to shake hands with me and say, "Thank you so much. Good night."

As they passed through the line some of the boys had shown me the purchases they had made in the near-by village—cherries and eggs and bottles of vino, and I was offered part of it all. One boy was deeply hurt because I would not take more than two of his eggs when he wanted to give me a full dozen.

Whatever other memories I may have of my work here, I shall never forget that night, the plateau stretching out under the North African sky splendid with stars, the dark shapes of the mountains crouching on the horizon, the vague blur of trucks scattered over the area, the little mounds on the ground where some of the men had already gone to sleep in their bed rolls, the glare of the headlights focused on the big kettle of coffee and the boxes of doughnuts, and the long line of eager, friendly boys from back home. My three-hour "shift" left me very weary, but it left me feeling that I should take off my hat to the "glamour girls" who do this kind of thing day after day, their smiles just as spontaneous and cheerful at 10 o'clock at night as at 10 in the morning.

By the end of June invasion restlessness was in the air and rumors were spreading fast and furiously. Day after day large formations of American bombers passed over our heads on the way to attack enemy installations in Sicily and Italy. On July 9, 1943, the invasion of Sicily began with the descent of Allied airborne troops and our patient load soon included casualties from Sicily. On August 17 the conquest of Sicily was complete; early in September the Fifth Army landed in Salerno and the British First Airborne Division occupied the naval base of Taranto. Within a few days we began to receive patients from Italy, the third major campaign the hospital had supported while based near Constantine. Early in October we were told the hospital would probably move at an early date; by the end of the month the last patient had been evacuated and the hospital was closed in preparation for the move.

It had been a long hot summer, as I wrote, with temperatures usually well over 100 during the day in the shade and up to 135 degrees Fahrenheit in the sun. When the *sirocco* was blowing in from the desert, it made housekeeping and office work much more difficult because it deposited layers of dust on everything. The sudden unexpected gusts of wind whirled papers off desks, blew supplies out of cabinets and even ripped letters out of typewriters. Tent ropes had to be tightened and the almost ceaseless flapping of the canvas soon caused frayed nerves and uncertain tempers.

I wrote home on July 3 that the wildlife in North Africa was certainly not what I'd expected, i.e. tigers and camels and huge snakes and scorpions! Although I did see camels quite frequently, the tigers and big snakes and scorpions never appeared. Instead we had many hungry grasshoppers who chewed holes in clothes and books, lots of little black biting bugs and

many ants who change their domicile every month or so and who have to be discouraged from moving their winter provisions of dead bugs into our tent! In addition there was a little brown mouse with pretty ears who lived under Irene Tobias' (my tentmate) cot, and I saw him for the first time yesterday when he came out for a late breakfast. There were also several rabbits who had discovered Irene's garden and who were having a lovely time eating the tops off her nasturtiums, much to her annoyance . . . and there are the flies which, according to posters and radio broadcasts spread diarrhea and dysentery and should be trapped, poisoned or swatted. So, while our wild life is not romantic, it keeps us busy trying to discourage its "friendly advances."

Church attendance doesn't seem to have been high on my list of priorities, partly because Sundays were generally just like weekdays with lots of work. In mid-July one of the enlisted men and I found what we thought was an Episcopal church that turned out to be a Methodist Episcopal one. (The soldier, Pfc. Orren Fox, was assigned to duty with the Red Cross and he was absolutely invaluable in the many ways he helped us and because of his unfailing cheerfulness.) We attended the service anyway and then went to the other extreme and attended Mass at the Roman Catholic Cathedral. A week later, after much telephoning, I learned that the British chaplain had Church of England services every Sunday. So I got up at six one Sunday morning and with my previous week's companion drove into Constantine. The services were held in a very small unadorned room with a plain wooden altar. There was a rack of fencing foils and masks on one wall, the floor was tile (and very hard and cold on the knees), and the benches just pieces of wood. I wrote home that

I got more real satisfaction out of the short simple service there than I did out of the colorful and dramatic service at the Cathedral. It was a coming home feeling to go through the familiar Order of Service and I hadn't really known just how much I'd missed it and how personally unsatisfactory I'd found the Army's Protestant services at the hospital. It was the first time I'd received Communion since I'd left Boston more than six months earlier and I was rather amazed how much it meant to me!

My official July monthly report gave a brief account of my varied job responsibilities; there seemed to be less real secretarial work so I was asked to help the social workers and at the end of the month did some pinch-hitting in the recreation department. Both these gave me more direct contact with the patients especially on the wards, which I enjoyed very much. I "made rounds" every day, covering each ward at least every third day, talking and joking with the men, filling requests for comfort articles, V-mail [the U.S. military mail system], EFM [Expeditionary Forces Mail] forms, writing occasional letters, looking at postcards or souvenirs or pictures of family and friends back home. I enjoyed it all very much—more so in the main than the difficult physical conditions, though even they were interesting, as my report made clear:

They told us when we first got here to remember that Africa was a cold country with a very hot sun. This is true enough, most of the year, but they forgot to mention that in July it stays hot even after the sun goes down. The Sirocco, hot and dust laden from the desert, makes housekeeping and office work more difficult with the layers of dust it deposits on everything and with sudden unexpected gusts of wind which whirl papers off desks, supplies out of cabinets, rips papers being typed and at times even threatens to bring the very tent down upon one's head. Tent ropes must be tightened, papers must be weighted down with books, or stones, or even elbows, and one must condition oneself to hear the telephone ringing above the ceaseless flapping of the tent fly. I must admit that there are times when despite the advantages and pleasures of tent life, I find myself wistfully longing for an office in an air-conditioned building, where nature can be kept at bay by walls and windows. However, these moods are rare and usually I enjoy the pyjama clad legs of the patients or the bare feet of the Arabs going past the rolled up sides of the tent, watching the shadows change on the cliffs across the valley and the clouds come and go in the intensely blue sky overhead. I think that it will be rather hard to adjust to city life again after the war, and that in spite of the advantages of four walls and a roof, I shall probably have a feeling of claustrophobia at first and remember with longing the freedom of our tents.

July brought variety to my job again. . . . One of the most exciting moments was when I was able to locate, in the nearby city, the twin brother of one of the patients. They had not seen each other for over a year and it was just luck and a couple of telephone calls that brought them together on this afternoon. The brother's outfit had just moved near here, and it was the merest chance that made me remember having heard his name mentioned by one of my friends. A call to my friend confirmed the matter, a call to the outfit, another call to the office where he was working at the moment, and half an hour later he was out here and the two of them, almost identical in appearance, were talking so fast and simultaneously that one wondered how they understood each other at all. The smiles on their faces and the twinkle in their eyes made me feel like a fairy godmother, and I'm sure I went around with a very self-satisfied expression the rest of the day. . . .

Several times during my ward rounds I had the opportunity to go into the prison wards, something I had not done before. I'd been a little curious as to my reaction to these men, but found I had no hostile feelings about it at all. They, too, were patients with needs which I would try to meet.

During the hot summer days, excursions to Philippeville, a nearby seaport (now called Skikda), were made as often as possible, sometimes on our days off for much-needed rest and recreation and sometimes for business of one sort or another. I wrote home on July 27 about one special trip which combined business and pleasure. I had persuaded my friends in the Signal Corps unit stationed there to give us some lengths of chicken wire to use as a backstop for our baseball diamond. So we took a two-and-a-half-ton truck down to pick it up, leaving quite early in the morning in order to make sure the seven of us would have enough time for the pleasure part of the trip.

Villages were just waking up, roosters crowing, and the people getting ready to go into market were filling their baskets with produce to sell. The flocks on the hillsides were stirring and sleepy shepherds lifted their heads as we went by, peering at us from under their hoods which kept half hidden their dark inscrutable faces. All young things seemed wide awake. Baby goats butted each other, lambs kicked up their heels, small burros wiggled their long ears and naked children ran out of doorways. We got to the top of the range of mountains between us and the sea and looked down into the sunlit valley ahead of us, the one behind us still shadowed in the half light of dawn. The sun ahead of us had been up at least an hour but the mists and clouds were still rising and made the more distant mountain peaks seem to be floating and disassociated from the valleys from which they were separated by the mist. Most of the hills were yellow or brown now, burned dry by the hot summer sun, but the olive groves were still a dark green. Along the road in several places the eucalyptus trees still filled the air with their clean fragrance, and the oleanders still marked in wandering lines of pink the banks of the now dry brooks. Early in the morning there seems to be more to smell than at other times; I suppose the dampness of the air has something to do with it. I could smell the warm earth, the sweetness of a flower that looks something like Queen Anne's Lace, fresh baked bread as we went by an Army bakery tent and many other unidentified smells, almost all of them pleasant. Later in the day the unpleasant smells came out and one can tell half a mile away when one is approaching a village!

As we got close to P . . . [Philippeville—in my letters I was careful for security reasons never to use place names], we began to meet people going in to market, riding donkeys or mules or bicycles, in carriages or on foot. There was a very picturesque Arab dressed in his best white robes, riding a really good horse, and solemnly carrying a big white umbrella with a green lining! It was wonderful.

The chicken wire was down on the beach so Gladys (the nurse who went with us) and I went swimming while the men cut it, rolled it and loaded it. That took only about half an hour so we all went to our "special" beach and spent the rest of the morning swimming and lying on the beach in the sun. . . . I rode home, again in the back of the truck, on top of the big rolls of chicken wire, with a blanket on top, very comfortable indeed.

There were other expeditions. A blind date I had toward the middle of July turned out not only to be nice but also a "good contact" as he was from the Medical Supply Depot and had occasional access to a jeep. He offered to take me to Timgad, where there are ruins from the sixth or seventh century. So we set off one day, on the three-hour drive through fascinating country. Riding in a jeep is almost as much fun as riding in the back of a truck and enables one to get quite a good view of everything. First, as I wrote on August 2:

We passed three or four salt lakes, water out in the middle but with a deep rim of salt around the edges that were shining and white in the brilliant sunshine like the rim of snow and ice on New Hampshire lakes at the beginning of winter. Then a bit of open plain with flocks of sheep and goats and herds of cattle watched over by Biblical shepherds. Then the hills came, mostly rocky ledges curiously eroded by the centuries so that all the edges were jagged and unexpected. We drove through a small pass and the hills changed completely with low scrubby trees and bushes appearing all over the tops. We passed at least a half dozen camel caravans, the supercilious creatures rolling along looking out of long-lashed eyes and slightly curling their upper lips over their teeth. They are really such silly-looking beasts but are reputed to have evil tempers and a nasty habit of biting when displeased.

It was threshing time and the Arab farmers were all busily engaged in separating the wheat from the chaff, usually with a couple of mules tied to a stake in the middle of the threshing floor and driven around in a circle, literally trampling out the wheat. Then it is all tossed into the air, the heavier kernels thus separating from the lighter chaff. A pretty sight but an obviously laborious and lengthy process.

I hadn't really expected to enjoy the ruins at "T" [Timgad] and had gone more from a sort of intellectual curiosity but I found them tremendously interesting. Our Arab guide had a white handkerchief on his head topped by a big straw hat. And of course the usual baggy trousers which, according to legend, are worn by all true believers because the Koran promised that when Mohammed came again he would be born of a man. The baggy trousers are supposed to ensure that if born suddenly, he wouldn't get hurt dropping to the ground!

The two main streets ran north–south and east–west with each gate named for the big city in that direction, i.e. C [Carthage], T [Tunis], B [Bizerte] and S [Sitif]. The big paving stones were worn in ruts from the wheels of the ancient Roman chariots. There was an elaborate system of drains as well as an aqueduct which brought water down from the mountains to the city. There were arcades along some of the streets and in the market place the stalls were marked with designs indicating the merchandise sold there: fish, wheat etc. The latrines had dolphins on the sides and the "house of ill repute" which the guide showed to Neale but not to me had, I understand, a design over the door that was unmistakable!!

I was so interested and even thrilled that a week later Neale and I went to Djemila, a bit longer drive than the one to Timgad but equally picturesque and fascinating. I was amused to see big advertisements of beverages popular in France painted on the sides of some of the houses in the little towns we passed through, DUBONNET and an occasional BYRRH. As I wrote home:

An Arab village is sometimes quite a collection of huts and hovels, and sometimes just a big house with its outhouses enclosed by a wall. The houses are made mostly of fieldstone with thick brush roofs, low doors and few windows, but I've seen some made of a sort of adobe like the Mexican huts. Chickens and children together scramble in the dust of the dooryard and wrinkled, tired women sit on the doorstep, while nearby in the farmyard the men direct the span of horses or mules attached to a center pole as they plod around and around trampling out the wheat . . . Except for early in the morning and late in the evening, the air is hot and heavy and dusty, the bright sunlight is almost oppressive on one's head and eyes, and the sky itself seems too near, weighing one down. How the people live there, I don't know. Many of the houses have no shade at all and at noon the sheep press tight up against the walls of the house, trying to squeeze into the narrow shadows. A few fortunate "villages" are near streams, now dried up to a muddy trickle but which in the rainy season must overflow their banks. Here the women and children are down at the edge of the puddles, washing clothes or playing in the water. The boys up to seven or eight usually wear no clothes at all but the little girls have some sort of covering, often so ragged that it seems a wonder they can keep it on at all, and so tattered that they would be better dressed without it! So near their homes and being of such a poor class, the women are often without their veils and dark outer dress. Some of the dresses are quite bright and gay, and it is a shock to see the old faces and toothless grins. They all look the same age, I don't know where the younger women are for one never sees them.

Those who live in the most fertile spots have little gardens and one can recognize melon patches and tomato plants and beans. And the ever-present fig tree of this part of the country. The figs are not quite ripe yet but the heat of the sun brings out their odor and one can tell around a corner when one is approaching a fig tree by the fragrance in the air. They make lovely deep pools of shade on sunbaked hillsides.

As we drove past, the children would come rushing out to watch us go by. They would wave at us and hold up their fingers in the "V" sign the soldiers have taught them, and yell "O.K., Joe, cigarette, chew gum, bon bon?" which they have also learned from the soldiers. The women are shy and just look, perhaps half-covering their faces as a gesture to modesty. The men stop their work to wave or salute us and I salute back, as much to amuse me as to please them. With all the waving that one does driving around here, I feel rather as though I were running for governor or something.

This is distinctly a grazing country. Huge flocks of sheep

and black goats and cattle roam the fields and roads, all in one big herd not separated as one would find back home. It makes driving slightly exciting for the silly creatures will run one way then reverse their tracks and run right back across the road. In addition to these animals, we saw tremendous herds of camels, some tucked into little valleys and some high against the skyline. Back here in the hills I saw my first nomad Arabs whose bright striped tents were pitched in the middle of the brownish yellow hill slopes, their flocks around them and their precious camels grazing in the background. I had read about them but never expected to see them. The tents are very low and made of striped rugs, probably camel hair. A few times we had to wait for the camels to lumber off the road, some of the little ones looking very long legged indeed.

We had been slowly but steadily climbing up all this time—suddenly we reached the top, rounded a curve and there beyond a valley were the most wonderful range of mountains, not jagged peaks but rounded tops furrowed and lined with deep creases looking something like a roll of beautiful brown velvet which had been tossed into hills and valleys. Any description of it would be most inadequate, and even photographs would not do it credit.

Half way down into the valley the ancient Roman city of Curcul [now called Djemila] sits on its own little hilltop, looking down the valley in front of it and up into the mountains surrounding it. It is a much bigger and better-preserved city than "T" [Timgad] which we went to before. The biggest part of it is fourth century A.D. but part goes back to the second century and part up to the fifth. It had a population of about 20,000 people. There are ruins of a Christian church with well-preserved vaults underneath and a baptismal font decorated with stone fishes and some of the mosaic still apparent on the bottom. There is the temple of Septimus Cerverus, 219 A.D. [more accurately Septimius Severus, I am now advised] and the Temple of Venus with marble and onyx from "P" [Philippeville] where we go swimming. Instead of storks as there were at "T", here there are pigeons nesting on top of the arches and in little corners of the stones. A great many stone tablets were still legible, if one can read Latin (I was amazed at how much I had forgotten) and it was interesting to notice the Hebrew influence in the shape of the letters. The temple of Jupiter had dungeons underneath it, with holes in the rock for chains to pass through. On the stone floor there are marks where the heavy doors scraped a quarter circle being opened and closed. The drains in the streets are shaped like a four-petal flower. And the public latrines, seating about twenty people, would probably cause a new "Specialist" to be written, Neale said [referring to Chick Sales's amusing book about privies]. One of the most complete buildings was the big gymnasium with hot and cold baths, private cubicles, steam baths, dressing rooms, exercise room and lovely big terrace in front with a wonderful view. The mosaic here is still present on the floor and on the walls. It gives one a queer feeling to be in a place that is so old and to think of all the people who came there and all the things that must have happened. One feels very small and insignificant and very much part of the passing parade.

Our guide spoke very little English, and much of it was profane from his experience with the soldiers and he was nowhere near as picturesque as the guide we had at T. He took us through the museum, which was interesting but seemed dead in comparison to the city itself. There were lots of statues, walls covered with mosaic, and showcases filled with tools, implements and dishes and such.

By this time we were both thirsty and hungry. At the top of the hill above the ruins was a little "Hotel" which looked cool and pleasant. We had heard that they would cook for you if you brought the food, so we expected to get only something to drink. The front of the house was shaded by trees and covered with vines; we went through a passage into a delightful courtyard roofed over with a grape arbor. The sunlight came through in patches, the big grape leaves keeping most of it out, and the heavy bunches of green grapes, not quite ripe, were almost translucent. There were two cats who wandered around under the tables, rubbing against the chairs in contented fashion, there was the singing of locusts and the gentle whisper of a breeze through the vines. The light was diffuse and green, like at the bottom of the sea with occasional bright patterned spots on the flagstones. Around the edges of the courtyard were pots of callas and oxalis (according to Neale; I wouldn't know). All in all, it was sleepy and cool and lovely. We sat at a little iron table and drank a slightly cool vin rosé, and didn't talk much, talking would have spoiled part of its charm.

At first we were the only people there, but as the afternoon wore on, more and more people came and we were joined by a Catholic chaplain whom we had talked to in the museum. He was very Irish, from San Francisco, and quite fun. The waiter took quite a fancy to me and said he would make us an omelette and salad for supper. So we drank some more *vin rosé* and ate a perfectly delicious omelette (three eggs apiece) and a very oniony tomato salad and a rather sour dark bread.

Time passed and reluctantly we decided we must leave. There was a spell to the place which we hated to break. But there was a long ride ahead of us, so we thanked the Padre— he had insisted on paying for the supper—and made our *adieux*. We took the long way back, delighting in the sunset and twilight and then the new moon and bright stars. Neale pointed out a group of stars called the River of Sighs, which was new to me. When is Guy Fawkes Day? As we passed a British camp, there was quite a display of fireworks in the hills. I wanted to make something exciting out of it, spies or distress signals or something but Neale spoiled it all by saying he thought it was Guy Fawkes Day.

Neale was wrong about that, as the English ditty reminds: "Please to remember / the Fifth of November / Gunpowder

39

Treason and Plot." In any case, I was quite ready for bed when I got back, as you can imagine.

I wrote home on August 18 about quite a different kind of trip when I was asked by one of our lieutenant colonels to do some interpreting for him.

[He] knew no French at all when he came over and has really made remarkable strides in learning it. He has made a number of friends among the local people, went boar hunting last spring with the Mayor of the next little town. Anyway, through some of his French friends he heard of a woman who had a badly injured leg, an old fracture which had been badly set at first, and whose doctor had been called away by the Army. She had been receiving massage in town, but the *masseur* had also left and she wanted advice. So Joe volunteered to go down and look at it and he took me along to interpret. It was an interesting visit, but I soon discovered that while my French may be adequate for social purposes, the specialized vocabulary covering X-rays, plaster casts, crutches, skin and bone and tendon grafts and transplants and so forth, had me completely buffaloed. However, we did remarkably well and Joe and I between us managed to understand her and to get our meaning across. Joe decided to bring the X-rays back to the hospital for an orthopedic man to look at. Then we decided to go and call on the Mayor and his family with, I must admit, the ulterior motive of hoping we would get an invitation to go horseback riding.

They are very pleasant people—mother, father, married daughter with small baby, younger daughter about [my younger sister] Joan's age named Josie, Anne and a son about twelve called Jeanot. We were invited up to their "apartment" which is the entire floor above the little cafe-bar on the main (and only) street. The windows in the back open into the stable yard and there is some of the to-be-expected odor in the house. The living room is typical enough of the family and the life and their class of society to be a stage-set. Sort of a golden oak living dining room set, a few very overstuffed chairs and everything covered with scarves and antimacassars and doodads. They served us anisette, which I cannot stand and which I had to drink to be polite, and we sat and talked and smiled for about an hour. And we got invited to go riding the next evening. Grandpa, the patriarch of the village, came to call too, so it was very much an evening *en famille*.

We went back a week later and this time we took with us the hospital's physiotherapist who had been a student under Dr. Arthur Watkins at Massachusetts General Hospital when I was working there. One of the boys from the physio department came too.

We had a perfectly hysterical two hours, as neither Lucy or the boy spoke any French and their attempts to teach "our" patient the correct way of walking with her crutches, the best exercises for her to do by herself, and so forth, were most amusing. I only wish Art could have seen it. I told Lucy I would have to write him about it, but perhaps one of you will see him and tell him. It was exciting too, to see how much more motion she had after her massage and how quickly she caught on to what they were showing her. From an ungainly, awkward cripple she became a potentially normal member of society again. Her amazement at the gentle massage was fun—apparently the style used here is the vigorous pounding Swedish school, and she couldn't get over the light stroking motions. It was a very satisfying experience.

Some of my letters home were written in our office tent during relatively quiet moments of the day. As I was typing the above I became aware of someone standing in front of my desk and looked up to see a patient with an armed guard behind him. Gave me quite a shock! I don't remember what it was that he wanted, probably a pack of playing cards or perhaps a toothbrush.

Another long letter described one of my days off when I spent a luxurious morning, going back to bed and reading for an hour after breakfast, puttering around my tent and washing all the clothes that the heavy storm had blown off the clothesline and buried in the mud. And then spending a quiet afternoon at the beach with three friends. Afternoons like that mended the tears and rents that the previous week had made in my disposition, peace of mind and tranquillity of spirit. Sometimes, I wrote, the holes are just "ladder runs," starting from a little snag and running down from there, involving other threads, and sometimes they are little moth holes of neglect, and sometimes big jagged "barn door" tears from quite heavy sharp encounters. That day I came back with most of them pretty well patched up and some even invisibly mended. In other words, a day off at the beach has very definite therapeutic value!

My letter home on August 24 tells of dinner with an Arab chief two days earlier:

Last spring, when we first got here, Joe Borg went boar hunting several times with the Mayor in the next village, some of his friends, and an Arab chief. From time to time this summer the chief has ridden up to the hospital on his best horse and dressed in his best clean cream-colored burnoose and white turban, bringing presents of melons or eggs or tomatoes. The last time he came he invited Joe to dinner and asked him to bring some friends. The two other doctors who had gone hunting with him were away on detached service, so Joe asked me and Mary Mock (my "boss") and Charlie Polan to go with him. He warned Mary and me that we might have to eat in the harem with the women, but that didn't discourage us at all.

The chief lived way back in the hills about ten miles back of the hospital on a narrow winding road which at times threatened to dwindle out entirely. We were a bit uncertain as to the exact locality of our host's dwelling and looked questioningly at each farm as we approached it, hoping for some sign that would indicate our expected presence. And sure enough, there were a series of small boys posted at the entrance to his road and at intervals up the road. The first one signaled madly to the second, who passed the signal on when he saw us coming and then climbed on the running board of our car to direct us in and out of the tall stacks of wheat to a place where we might park. The signaling resulted in our host coming out to meet us and in the banishment of the women from the farmyard to the safe confines of their own part of the house.

The chief was strikingly dressed in a plaid shirt open at the neck, a pair of riding breeches which came midway on the calf of his leg and which were pulled down enough at the waist to show a couple of inches of his treasured white undershorts(!), no socks, brown and white sport shoes and his white turban. It was really something. He insisted on taking us on a "grand tour" of his farm before we went in, showing us the tremendous amount of wheat he had harvested, pointing out the *figues de barbaries* (prickly pears to you), the big melon patch, the miles and miles of farmland all around that belonged to him, the cattle and sheep and goats on the slopes of the hills, and the beautiful view to the north. His farm was on the top of a hill and the view really was superb: miles of rolling hills covered with wheat fields and the mountains ringing us in on the horizon. (Mary and I were certainly glad we had worn clean white shoes, the way he unconcernedly led us over piles of manure and through the fields!)

We were then escorted through the muddy, haphazardly cobbled outer courtyard, through a low archway into the inner courtyard and thence into the house. The room in which we were entertained was fairly small with only one window rather high in the wall. There was the door by which we came in, a door to the left of that with a pink silk curtain shutting it off, a steep stairway to the second floor, a blue curtained recess with shelves on which some of the china was kept and some of the food—in fact, I think there was an

43

opening into the kitchen there for I am sure some of the hot food came out of the recess—and a cupboard where the rest of the china, the bread, the honey and the grapes were kept. There was a table in the middle of the room and five chairs, and that was all. The floor was tile, there were beams across the ceiling and everything was whitewashed, so it seemed quite clean. We were offered anisette or beer—we all took the latter—but our host did not drink at all. Good Mohammedans don't drink, which I had forgotten. He spoke quite good French, by the way, and his brothers speak a little, but all the rest of the family manage to speak only Arabic. He tried to teach us several words, assuring us that it was very easy, but we were not apt pupils. He was much better at learning the English words we pronounced for him.

At first Hassin, our host, was not going to eat with us, saying that he preferred to serve us and would eat later, but we persuaded him that we would be honored by his presence at table with us. We started out with a perfectly delicious thick soup with meat and vegetables and much seasoning in it. Then came a meat dish with big chunks of tender boiled mutton and little meatballs of some sort, again highly spiced. We thought this was probably the main course but fortunately, just as we were about to take seconds, the next course was brought on and we were able to stop just in time. This course consisted of huge thick lamb chops, the first I had had in many, many months and a whole chicken. The chops were wonderfully prepared with something like parsley and a little onion on top and cooked just right. The chicken was good but not unusual. There were also hard-boiled eggs but we pretended to ignore them and he forgot to urge them on us until it was too late. By this time we were getting rather full and hoped the meal would take a downward curve from then on. But no, the next course was couscous, that sort of half-cooked white cornmeal I told you about before, with a peppery sauce. This hurdle safely negotiated, they brought on fruit. All during the meal we had been eating the native bread of which we had two kinds. It is baked in big plate-like slabs, about a foot and a half in diameter. The raised bread is about two inches high and the unleavened bread, which is made with butter and is fairly short, is only about half an inch thick. The latter is more like a biscuit than bread, but they are both very good and the sort of thing that you just go on taking one more bite of.

The first part of dessert was pears, both prickly pears and ordinary ones. The prickly pears were wonderful, completely unlike anything I had ever eaten before, so I cannot describe them to you. The other pears were a little hard and grainy but good. Then we had two kinds of melon, served one at a time so you didn't have a choice, you had to eat both! Watermelon and honeydew, both extremely good, but we were all so full at this point that we felt our eyes must be bulging. We asked Hassin if this was the way he ate all the time and he grinned and said it was not, usually they had only one meat course, but he hadn't wanted us to go home and tell our friends that we hadn't been well fed at his house, and he wanted us to have plenty to talk about when we got back to the States! After the melon we had both purple and green grapes, the biggest and best I had ever eaten, and dates. And then he brought on little honeycakes and, at last, the coffee. With obvious pride, he put the sugar bowl on the table too. Not only is it extremely difficult to get sugar over here, but the bowl was in the shape of a setting hen, and was made of milk glass. There were sugar tongs also. Really quite quite. The coffee cups were also things of great joy to him and they were very pretty. The coffee was thick and very bitter unless sugar was added and then he put in some *L'eau d'orange* which smelled a little like hair tonic but which added a very nice extra flavor. It was all I could do to find room for the coffee, but I somehow managed, while frantically trying to remember just where I had put those bicarb of soda tablets that Walter had given me on the boat!

In spite of the language difficulties, the conversation had

been pretty general throughout dinner. Mary speaks a pretty good convent French and Joe gets along amazingly well, but Charlie knows very little. Yet somehow he manages to understand and be understood. He says it is intuition, and we tell him it is because he is a psychiatrist and used to sort of mind reading! Hassin told us that he was the oldest of nine brothers, three of whom lived there on the same farm, Hassin and two younger ones. As far as we could gather, they each have three wives! The two brothers waited on us and in one corner of the room a whole crowd of children and cousins or something stood and watched us. At first they had been too timid to do anything more than peek in the window, hastily withdrawing when we looked up at them, but gradually they grew used to us and came right into the same room with those strange women who actually eat at the same table with the men, and go around with their faces all uncovered! I felt rather like something in the zoo.

Coming through the barnyard, we had noticed and admired some beautiful large white turkeys, the first we had seen over here. And now, as the meal was slowly drawing to a close, Hassin began to gather gifts for us to take home. During the last ten minutes of our coffee drinking, melons had been arriving, being presented to him for approval and then piled in the corner. Next came a basket of about three dozen eggs, to which he added the hard-boiled ones on the table which he had forgotten to press on us. He rushed upstairs and got a pencil so he could indicate which were cooked and which were not. And then, to our open-mouthed amazement, in came a fellow with one of the turkeys! A simply huge one, still alive too. Mary said she was certainly grateful that I had not admired a cow or a goat! We were so overcome that we couldn't say anything, so Mary finally came to the rescue and said it was just like Christmas, wasn't it? That confused Hassin until she explained about presents and things at Christmas. Then, curious, we asked if they had a holiday too, celebrating the birth of Mohammed. It appears they do and for some reason the day advances ten days every year. It is in the spring, now. Hassin still seemed curious about something and finally asked who our prophet was, whose birth it was we celebrated at Noël? Mary, a little astonished, said our prophet was Jesus Christ. Hassin's mouth made an O in surprise and he exclaimed, "*Ah, comme les français!*" and he turned in excitement to tell the people behind him in Arabic what we had said. Mary said afterwards that she had a hard time to keep from laughing, that apparently the Americans had such a reputation for being different from everybody else that the Arabs thought, of course, they had a different prophet. She thought our stock was lowered a bit when they learned that we shared such an important thing as a prophet with the French, whom they don't like at all. (Hassin assured us that after the war he was coming to America.)

We finally succeeded in making our farewells and started to go out the door, one of the brothers bearing a lamp to light our way and all the melons and the eggs and the turkey divided up among about ten small children to carry to the car. Just as I reached the door, Hassin made a sudden exclamation and almost pushed me back into the house, so I collided with all those behind me. I thought some of the women must have gotten loose and he was hastening to put them back under cover, but no, in a minute he reappeared with a small baby. My first thought was that this was a present too, but he merely wanted medical advice about the child's eyes which were badly inflamed and crusted along the lid margin and slightly swollen. Joe looked at the baby for a minute; then Hassin disappeared and came back with another one, whose eyes were even more swollen. It was apparently a bad conjunctivitis; Charlie said if it were trachoma more than two would have it. I hope he is right. I think Joe will take them some Argyrol [a patent silver-protein compound] next time he goes.

We crossed the courtyard in the dark, veering suddenly to

right or to left as the dark shape of a sleeping cow rose up in front of us. (Earlier, when the cattle came home at sunset, one of them had to be dissuaded from coming in to join the party. We heard a loud moo and looked up to see the creature halfway into the room!) Let me tell you, a cow lying down looks awfully big in the dark! We finally got us and our loot arranged in the car, with the turkey lying on the floor at Mary's feet, its head nearest Joe at her request! The night was very dark indeed and the tops of these hills are something like the moors, it all looks the same and the road blends right into the fields. We thought we knew the way home and turned down Hassin's offer of a guide, but we got turned around and ended up in some other Arab's front yard, arousing a pack of very angry dogs and having two Arabs utter piercing whistles as they descended on us. They spoke no French but we mentioned the name of the town we wanted and by gestures and much guttural noises they showed us the way to go. And then we ended up again back at Hassin's! Apparently he had watched our lights and saw we were lost and had posted a guide to help us. Finally we got on the right road and safely back home, where we staggered exhausted to bed.

We are having a picnic tonight to eat the turkey; he got out this morning and the boys in the utility shop, where I had parked him, called me up in a frenzy this morning just as I got down to work, so I took [Pfc. Orren] Fox and we went over to catch him. Must have made quite a sight, me chasing that turkey around and under ambulances down at the motor pool. We had quite a crowd cheering us. Poor turkey, he had seen the lovely peacock that lives at the next farm and had escaped to make friends with it. We finally caught him, and right now he is being stuffed or perhaps he is already in the oven.

In my official Red Cross report for August I omitted all of the above, needless to say, commenting instead on the more usual and regular aspects of my job, such as writing letters, settling arguments with the help of the one remaining office dictionary, and even copying poems. Some of these poems had been written by soldiers while on active duty, but others were the result of long hours in bed at the hospital. Good or often quite bad, they were obviously therapeutic in the expression and release of emotions. It was very difficult for me to know just what to say as I gave the neatly typed poem back to the proud author. I finally hit on saying wonderingly, "And is this really the very first poem you've ever written?!" That, I found, satisfied them without offending my New England conscience.

In early September we called on our Arab friend Hassin again, taking Argyrol for the babies' eyes. He was very cordial but apologetic because he could not offer us what he considered appropriate hospitality. The month of fasting, Ramadan, had just begun, during which time Moslems do not eat, drink or smoke from sunrise to sunset, these times being determined by whether one can (at sunrise) or cannot (at sunset) distinguish a white thread from a black. A cannon is fired in town to announce the end of the day. When I lived in Turkey many years later with my husband and our children, I was glad I had had this earlier introduction to the custom.

Italy was invaded by the Eighth Army on September 3, 1943, which was exciting news indeed, and the surrender of Italian troops on September 8 gave further strength to the rumors of a move in the not-too-distant future. The days grew shorter as daylight-saving time came to an end and the weather was noticeably cooler and at night, quite cold.

In early October, I wrote about a long-anticipated trip through the dramatic gorge of the Rummel River with our Warrant Officer Ray Kaufman:

It was quite a hike but well worth the effort. At the entrance were two Arab boys washing some sheepskins, very freshly killed I should say. They were holding them under a small waterfall—I tried to take a picture of them, but I don't believe it came out very well. Farther up there was a little girl, dressed in a pink dress with a blue sweater, who was fishing with her grandfather, a bearded, white-haired Frenchman. She stood on a rock, perfectly reflected in the still water below her, and while we watched, she actually caught a fish. Just a little one, but it was very exciting. Grandfather helped her take it off the hook, but she put it in the creel herself and even rebaited her hook. I was most impressed. And what made the whole scene so striking, was the tremendous height of the dark looming cliffs behind her and the cave-like feeling the high rock arch gave to the place. There were maidenhair ferns growing in the rocks and swallows nesting on the face of the cliff, darting in and out. Quite a place.

On Wednesday September 8th, the hospital admitted a little French girl for a brain tumor operation. It had taken weeks to get all the necessary permission from all the Army officials, but it was finally arranged. Her family was from Rouen, but had moved over here for the duration, her father being an officer in the French Army. Jane was a very bright and intelligent child, about ten years old. She and her parents spoke no English, and the medical officers speak very little French. So I was called in as official interpreter. It was one of the most interesting things I have ever done, as I was present for all the consultations and examinations. The parents had brought with them the records of examinations and treatments in French hospitals, and I had to paraphrase all that for the doctors, then there was a period of questioning the parents, then various examinations of the child, including a neurological exam by a visiting fireman, a well-known New York neurosurgeon who did the first assist for the operation. Jane had had so many of these examinations before that she knew all the answers almost before the questions were asked.

Thursday was one of the most hectic days I have ever had. Mary was sick, Irene and Buff were away for a couple of days at a conference (yes, even here in Africa!) so Fran and I ran the whole Red Cross business for twelve hours straight. And besides Red Cross I had my little French girl to look after. But I enjoyed it all. Seems like the busier things are and the more hectic, the better I like it. Silly sort of a way to be, isn't it? Friday, Mary was back at work, which was just as well, as Jane took up a lot of time. There was another neurological exam and an ophthalmological exam, both of which we enjoyed immensely, making a game out of it. Then Friday night they cut her lovely hair off and shaved her head. She didn't like this at all, but I sat on the floor in front of her and we played with her doll and ate Life Savers and her mother brought some beer (which the child loves) and then we sang French nursery songs together. How I wished I could remember more of them, but on the whole I did pretty well and the two-hour procedure went off without any tears. She behaved remarkably well during the whole of her stay here, and I was equally impressed with the behavior of her parents, who had none of the to-be-expected emotionalism about it, and never let the child guess by any word or look or tenseness that they were worried half to death. She thought she was going for a new kind of X-ray, and was not in the least apprehensive.

By Friday night I was so worked up about the whole thing, and I hadn't been feeling well all week, had awful headache all the time, that I didn't go to bed until three in the morning. Then I slept only a couple of hours and was up and back with Jane again at 6:30. I went to surgery with her and reassured her and held her hand until she was under. Then they gave me a mask and let me stay for the operation. I couldn't see the whole thing as I had to go back to the office for part of the morning, but I saw most of it and Charlie stood beside me most of the time and told me what they were doing, so it was quite educational as well as interesting. Three of the French doctors from town who were interested in the case came out too so there was quite a gallery. It was extremely long, about four and a half hours, but it was quite successful. They were not able to remove all of the tumor, but a large part of it, and the child should live much longer and a much more normal life than if it had not been removed. I had the pleasure of finding the parents afterwards and telling them how well the whole thing had gone. Even then there was none of the effusiveness and emotion that I had expected.

My headache was much worse by Sunday, so I reported to Sick Call and was put in the hospital. They had a lovely time all week, doing all sorts of tests and fancy examinations, only to discover, just as I was better and they were going to let me go home, that I had Flexner's Dysentery! Quite a letdown, as I know they were thinking of meningitis and all sorts of things like that. Well, I got a two weeks' rest, which came in handy. And now I'm out again and feeling fine, but my alcoholic tolerance is very low, and even a drink of scotch which I had the other night didn't taste very good. Isn't that a sad state of affairs? Officially back to work full time the 28th of September.

The weather now is just like those lovely October days at home. Cold nights and crisp days, wonderful just to be alive in. Rumors are being born every minute—we are all very tired of this location and we're all of us hoping that the events in Italy will influence our future, soon.

Friday night last week the Welsh Guards came out to sing for us. Reminded me of "How Green Was My Valley" with the lovely Welsh voices in that. Good-looking chaps too— they say it is the Welsh Guards who are on duty around Buckingham Palace in peacetime, you know "They're changing guard at Buckingham Palace, Christopher Robin went down with Alice . . ."

Early in October, Mary Mock was given orders for her

transfer to Oran as the Red Cross Regional Hospital Supervisor, and Irene Tobias was transferred to work in a psychiatric hospital. So the parameters of my job changed once more. I got off to a good start by having a party for the patients in the mental ward.

I was scared to death and shaky with stage fright, but the party was a big success. The ward is one of the Nissen huts with two "isolation" rooms for the worst patients and about sixteen beds in the open part. We invited all the other patients on the psychiatric service who were in other parts of the hospital, and there must have been 30 or 40 men there, a couple of nurses, the ward boys and the chief of service, my friend Charlie. We played Bingo, which is an unfailing success anywhere at any time, and you would have been much amused to hear me master-of-ceremonies-ing the whole affair. Then a couple of patients said they had a show they wanted to put on, and they entertained us for half an hour with some quite amusing skits. I think they must have been show people in civilian life because of the ease with which they did it. Then we had a couple of boys from the detachment come and play the guitar for us and I even got some of the boys to sing a few songs, but the enthusiasm was not very great, and some of our "guests" began to drift away. So I decided it was time to eat—and the party quickly revived with hot cocoa and graham cracker sandwiches made with peanut butter. Being with them made me realize even more clearly how narrow is the line between sanity and insanity. Of course, many of these patients were not really crazy, most of them were anxiety and/or neurosis cases but even the craziest didn't seem as crazy as some of my friends!

One big event since I wrote you last was the time I covered an evacuation train which was transferring some of our patients to another hospital. Two of us go to the train and, talking with almost every patient on it, give cigarettes and matches enough for the trip, hard candy, playing cards and a small amount of reading material. It is an exhausting job but lots of fun. Saying goodbye at any time is emotionally exhausting, but when you multiply that by many score, all you are fit for is to go to bed for a couple of hours. This particular time both of the social workers and both of the recreational workers were unable to cover the job, so Fox and I did the job ourselves—I was the social worker and Fox the recreation. It was an English day, soft and foggy with occasional inconsequential showers. The train was a combination of old and dilapidated continental second-class coaches and "40 and 8" cars, [so called because French authorities in World War I designated these cars for either 40 men or 8 horses]. The litter patients were loaded into the 40-and-8s, the litters swung in tiers of three, which didn't give much headroom if one wanted to sit up! Some of the men had parts of uniforms, shirts or pants or sometimes both, or pillows or sheets, of course, or just the litter to lie on and a blanket over them. Before the train pulled out, it had gotten quite dark and the attendant for each car lit kerosene lanterns which he hung from a ceiling hook, leaving them to swing gently back and forth in the breeze. It didn't give much light and the corners of the car were as dark as ever, and you could not recognize the faces of the men in the litters, but the white casts and fresh bandages shone dimly. I clambered in and out of the cars, with a wastebasket full of cigarettes and matches, trying to fill individual requests for Luckies or Camels and saving the unpopular Raleighs for the end. Fox had *Stars and Stripes* [the Army newspaper] and the playing cards, and then we came back later with big boxes of hard candy, individual paper sacks of it for the litter patients and boxes to put in the compartments of the ambulatory. Willing hands always reached down out of the boxcar doors to pull me up, and Fox would get down first and catch me as I jumped out, as the "step" was a good three feet off the ground. (Fox said that the next day any number of detachment boys had offered to buy his job, as they thought they would enjoy the part of helping me down out of the boxcars! Fox gallantly said he would not sell for any price!)

The litter patients taken care of, we moved on to the ambulatory patients who were being jammed into tiny compartments. The train smell was a familiar one, smoke, stale air, old cigarettes and the musty plush on the seats. Here, too, there were no lights, except for an occasional flashlight or a dim light in the vestibule or halfway down the corridor alongside the compartments. I went up and down, saying goodbye to special friends, telling the men to give our greetings to the Red Cross in the next hospital, answering questions and exchanging jokes. I almost got mobbed when I decided to vary the routine by calling out "Chicken sandwiches, ham sandwiches, ice cream and soft drinks." They practically threw me off the train. But at least it created a slight diversion. Before I left, they started serving hot coffee and the clouds of steam from the big pitchers as they were carried under the light looked like a scene from an Alfred Hitchcock picture. A bunch of the officers who were leaving dragged me into their compartment and loaned me a big tin mug so that I could have some too, so I perched on the edge of the seat arm and had a moment's respite from my labors.

The whole affair was curiously unreal, a scene in a movie thing. It was dramatic and moving and good "copy," extremely tiring, and one of the most fascinating and interesting couple of hours I have spent in a long time. Fox and I limped home after the job was finished. I had a date to go to the movies with Charlie but I joined him at the club, had a drink and was too tired to even talk, so I went home to bed. Irene did another train the other day, the afternoon before a dance, and came home to rest a bit before the party. She went to sleep, I woke her up twice and each time she was too tired to get up and went right back to sleep. When I got home at 12:30 she was still asleep on top of the bed with all her clothes on. Mary did an early morning train once, came home about nine A.M. and, lying down for a few minutes before coming down to the office, fell asleep and slept the rest of the morning. And Buff came home after a train job too tired to clear off her bed and went to sleep on the floor! Physically the job isn't all that tiring, it is emotionally that it wears you out.

October was also Christmas shopping time. In my official report for the month I wrote:

October has seemed to come to an end almost before it properly began. It was one of our busiest months, busy not only with the ordinary day-by-day routines but with interesting and satisfying small jobs and sudden demands on our time and energies. One of these sudden demands came from the Quartermaster who wanted our help in having the Army Exchange Service for Christmas shopping brought to the attention of every bed patient, a job which could easily have taken a week or two but which we had to complete in 48 hours. The combination of Christmas shopping so early and so far away from home sounded ludicrous to many and my announcement in each ward was greeted with laughs and derisive comments, but on second thought they remembered mother, wife, sweetheart and children—and sometimes as a reluctant afterthought, mother-in-law—and realized that it was about time to do something about Christmas presents. Frequently, after the "we cannot guarantee anything" policy of the Army was explained to them, they decided to send a money order with a shopping list to a friend at home, but even if they did not take advantage of the shopping service, I felt that the time talking with them was well spent as it brought to light a dormant need. If they did put in an order, many of them wanted help in the seemingly insoluble problem of what to give a woman, which perfume would she like, or what kind of flowers. Some expressed an almost bitter lack of interest and said they were not giving any presents this year; some wanted to know if there was any way they could send the candy to themselves; but the best of all were those who smiled and said they did not need to order their gifts now, as they would be home for Christmas. In a hospital probably, but a hospital in North America not one in North Africa or in a foxhole in Italy.

The steady rain, the mud, our floppy raincoats, hats and boots, and the chilly ward tents . . . it all should have made Christmas seem very unreal indeed but somehow thinking about it and talking about it, picking out a panda for a baby or a manicure set for a wife, made it seem like December, not October, and it was all I could do to keep from wishing the patients a Merry Christmas as I left the ward.

I did much of my own Christmas shopping in town and proudly noted in my journal on October 15 that I had mailed them all. A very wise activity in view of the fact that we had had definite word about moving, probably by the end of the month.

There were several large evacuation trains from the front whose patients had to be cared for while our unit prepared to leave, as tents were struck and some equipment was packed, ready for shipment to some as yet unknown destination. A new Red Cross worker, Anne Aldridge arrived. Various farewell parties were given and last, but far from least, I was at last able to get travel orders for Fran and me to go on leave to Tunis. On October 31, I wrote home about one final episode:

One of the best stories of the moment is about my little Italian beau who works in the bakery here at the hospital (the organization of an army outfit like this hospital is really something. We are pretty nearly self-sufficient—our own bakery, generate our own electricity, build our own furniture, even a tailor and of course a barber. It is most impressive when one sits down to think about it, but mostly we just take it for granted). Anyway, to get back to Vincenzio or whatever his name is. He isn't a very big fellow but he has big lovely dark eyes, dark curly hair and a little dark moustache. He speaks a little English but not much. I met him first one day as he was walking across the area carrying a big tray full of fresh and very fragrant hot biscuits. I smiled at him and said "*Bueno*" pointing at the biscuits. He smiled back and replied, "*Si, bueno,*" and that, I thought, was the end of that. But no, later in the afternoon I looked up from my typewriter to see him standing smiling in the doorway, and my answering smile brought a perfect torrent of Italian upon my head. He was much disappointed to learn that I did not speak it after all, and took over in broken English. The conversation ran something like this: "You like biscuit, no? Today boss no give me biscuit. You like doughnuts, yes? Tomorrow, maybe I get doughnuts bring to you." I assured him that indeed I did like both biscuits and doughnuts and that it was very nice of him to think of me but that really he must not bother. We parted with much smiles and "*grazie.*" He was as good as his word and the next day, after first coming by the tent to make sure I was there, he brought me eight fresh doughnuts. The following day he again stopped in to find out if I liked apple pie. Of course I said yes and ten minutes later he brought me a great big piece of pie! He had asked me earlier if I could give him some cigarettes but I explained to him that those were only for the patients. However, after the apple pie I felt that something should be done, so with the help of an interpreter, I gave him a pack of cigarettes, explaining that it was from me, not from the Red Cross, sort of from one friend to another. He understood, I think. The climax came today when he arrived with a little paper bag and handed it to me, saying that he was giving me his heart. I opened it and he had made a big heart out of baking-powder biscuit dough and put his initials on it! I am really quite touched by his attentions, although I am holding my breath to see what form it will take next! The Italians all seem to like me—perhaps I am the type that appeals to them, or something.

In a hurriedly scrawled V-mail letter written the next day, I apologized for my unusual brevity by explaining that we were suddenly forced by the really torrential rains to move all the Red Cross stuff out of our tents into one of the Nissen huts which, we learned later, we were to share with the two chaplains. Our desks and the piano were at one end and the altar at the other… one automatically lowered one's voice as one walked in! I almost expected my little Italian bakery beau to cross himself and genuflect when he came in to see me the next day bringing me some "pie-cake," another big biscuit heart, bigger this time with two little hearts superimposed on it and he also brought a piece of spice cake and some pineapple-upside-down cake!

One soon learns that with the Army it is always "hurry up and wait." So I had plenty of time out at the airport on November 3 to write the following:

Well, maybe I will have a chance to finish this letter to you and then again maybe I won't. It is now eleven o'clock in the morning, and I have been up since four thirty. My leave officially started this morning but I am, as the Army says, "sweating out my transportation." I crept out of bed in the cold dark night, took a very desultory sponge bath (fortunately I found some warm water), finished packing my suitcase and dressed in the warmest clothes I could find, stumbled down the gravel paths through the quiet and sleeping hospital, to the Detachment Mess where to my joy I found that they were making pancakes for breakfast. I coaxed a plateful off the cook plus a cup of coffee and perched on the edge of a table to eat my breakfast. Then back to the tent for a last combing of the hair, and so off to the air field in an ambulance. There were five of us, and it was a quiet journey, with all of us still half asleep. The clouds were beginning to lift and the sun to tip their edges with pink just as we got out here. It had been such a wet and heavy night that for a while

59

we were afraid that all flights might be canceled. We checked in with our travel orders, which it had taken all the wiles of a siren plus the tiny bit of official business we invented to obtain, and we went over to the officers' mess for a second breakfast. I find that in moments of stress such as this the best thing to do is to eat often. However, once I get up in that plane, if ever, I may disagree with that finding. I'll let you know.

After this second breakfast, fried eggs this time, we came back to the field and had the disheartening experience of having one plane load and take off without us. One by one they called the names of those lucky ones, who had some sort of priority I guess, gave them those precious bits of paper which entitled them to get on the plane; bit by bit they loaded in the luggage and the mail, closed the doors and took off without us. Right up to the last minute I hoped that they would find another place and let me go, or at least let one of us go. But no. And now here we are, sitting in the sun on the strip of gravel in front of the tiny adobe hut which comprises the flight office. Four other nurses have joined us and we are each amusing ourselves in our own way. For a little while we got two of the young pilots who were lounging around to use the heavy guard rope as a jump rope and they turned for us as we did Teddy Bear and all the other fancy things brought from the dim memories of our childhood days. Tiring of that we climbed all over a tiny fighter plane that had just come in and one of the girls who knew the pilot very well got a ride—the plane is built for just one person and the pilot had to sit in her lap! My heart was in my mouth as I watched it come off the ground. It looked so laden down and I was so afraid that it would not get off, or that once off, it would do a nose spin or something. But they got off, flew around for ten minutes and came back again, none the worse for their crazy stunt. Must have been his red hair which brought them good luck.

I was content to sit in the sun and start a pair of red socks for half an hour or so, but soon all that warm underwear and sweaters and my slacks made the sun seem much too warm, so I smiled at the boys behind the desk and asked permission to use their typewriter. They have adopted me as mascot or something now, gave me the best typewriter saying that they wanted to make me as happy as possible as I would probably be here for some time. But not more than two or three days, they assured me! It is kind of fun for a bit though, the cool hut with a big window to my right through which I can watch the never-ceasing activity on the field. The day has completely cleared now, except for a few heavy white clouds on the horizon and hanging low on a few of the mountains at the rim of the valley. I am as dumb about planes as I am about cars, in fact the only way I can tell a plane from a car is that one is in the air and one is not. But I can tell that there are all sorts and types of planes here, all sizes and shapes. Probably just as well I don't know the different kinds, for even if I did, I am sure that the censor would not appreciate my listing them here. Oh well they are pretty anyway and as long as it flies, I don't much care what kind comes along and takes me up and off!

In spite of numerous phone calls to any and everyone I could think of who might have some influence, we were still at the airport by early afternoon when the hospital called to tell us to return to base. I finished my letter back in my tent, wondering whether to clear off my cot or sleep on the floor!

We learned the next day that one of the reasons we had been called back was to pack up all our personal belongings in preparation for a move into more waterproof buildings during our absence. As I wrote later, it was a very hectic twenty-four hours:

Until one begins to pack, one never realizes just how much stuff, and I do mean stuff, one has accumulated. It is simply incredible, and even after I had loaded down the little French boy who works in our officers' club with all sorts of things, such as soap, matches, straw baskets, and so forth, the size of my bedroll was appalling. I do not see how I can throw away anything else, yet I don't see what I have that makes it so big. There are all my Red Cross uniforms, of course, and then on top of all that there are all the G.I. clothes which we really need. Of course, I do have a year's supply of such things as soap and so far we have been able to purchase a bar a week at the P.X., but you do not dare stop buying or start throwing away because there is no way of telling when the P.X. supply will cease.

Anyway a frantic full day got me all packed. I folded up my cot so as to have room on the floor of my tent to roll the bedroll. (Luckily it was sunny all day but early in the evening the heavens opened and the rains descended in torrents. The electricity was off, and it was rather weird by candlelight.) So I slept on the floor on my bedroll. It was much more comfortable than I had anticipated, but then I was so tired that I think I could have slept almost anywhere without too much trouble. Once more we got up in the early, cold gray dawn, stumbled down to breakfast at 5:30, and once more drove out to the airport. At seven the weather was fairly promising, with suggestions of a sunrise, but by eight it had closed in and by the time we had finished our second breakfast, it was raining. We sloshed out to the Air Transport Office and sat around for several hours—rather I went out there and promised the others that I would call if there seemed to be any chance of clearing out. They preferred to stay in the relatively warmer officers' mess. I had made some good friends among the enlisted men the day before and I thought that if we had a really long wait, it would be wiser not to stick too much together. I set up my own typewriter this time and did a little leftover office work, then typed a few paragraphs on my impressions of the office there and the weather and the people. The place looked very much like what I think a dugout must have been like in the last war. It is an adobe hut, nothing but a clay dirt floor, and the night before the rains had been so heavy that the office part was flooded and there was a water line three inches up the wall. In the waiting room there were still big puddles and all the baggage had to be stacked in one dry corner. It was cold enough so that one's breath rose in a white cloud in front of one, and the disconsolate and patient passengers sat huddled in their coats, as close to each other as possible. Back of the counter where the boys and I were, the ten of us amused ourselves in different fashions. One boy was playing solitaire, two played checkers, one tended the Victrola which ground out over and over the same three records, one boy curled up on a table with his head on a parachute and slept away the cold and weary hours, three others leaned against the counter and told stories or argued about the relative merits of various types of planes. One thing that I did, after I finished typing, was to write two extremely corny poems for one boy who wanted a love poem to send to his wife and another one as sort of a general Christmas greeting. They were the love-dove, moon-soon, night-bright sort of thing, but he was as pleased as if Alfred Noyes had written them for him.

From time to time all of us would casually get up and stroll over to the window to see what the weather was doing. I don't believe there is any place as wet or as dismal or as gray as an airfield in the rain. The two planes outside the big window were blotted out from time to time by an extra heavy squall and the rest of the time they could just barely be seen, dripping from the wings and the propellers and the nose, standing in big puddles in a sea of red mud. One look sufficed, and we would stroll back to whatever we were doing.

We finally left the next morning in a bomber, the only flight cleared for departure that day as the field was socked in shortly after we took off. It was an incredible ride and one of the most exciting things I've done in an exciting life. I had the earphones on most of the way, and we listened to some music from Radio-France part of the way but the fun was just before we landed when they were calling in for landing directions. It was just like the movies! For a while we flew over a mile high, way above the clouds which were below us in white fluffy puffs. We saw a complete circle rainbow with a shadow of the ship in the middle. We flew right through the clouds and it felt like being in the middle of a down puff. It rained and the rain streamed off the curved window in front of us and the ship tossed up and down. We flew low over fields and villages, low over the water for a bit, then up and over some mountains. When we were in the clouds it was quite cold, but when we got up high in the sunshine, it was warm and quiet and peaceful and the world and war seemed far away indeed. It was hard to remember that this ship had seen much that was not quiet and peaceful. Flying is certainly something that I am going to want to do after the war. Letting someone else fly probably, but I might even get around to doing some of it myself. I hate to drive cars, but I think flying a plane might be quite different. Not as much danger of bumping into another plane, anyway.

As if flying to Tunis in a B-25 bomber wasn't exciting enough, on Sunday, November 7, the day after I arrived, I received a message that my father, Spencer Phenix, was in Algiers en route, as I learned later, to see Alex Kirk, the consul general in Cairo. I still have vivid memories of visiting the Kirks when I was growing up in Washington and my father was an assistant to the undersecretary of state. His work then--as well as later when we lived in New York, and during World War II and in the postwar years--occasioned many trips abroad, but I don't remember being much interested in knowing where he went or why. As he kept none of his personal papers, I have not been able to check possible reasons for this trip to Cairo or a later one to Madrid where we met again.

I spent the entire afternoon trying to get either to Bizerte where my orders were or Algiers without orders (not a recommended activity in wartime!). Finally I got orders to fly to Bizerte on Monday, and then on to Algiers on TDY [temporary duty] orders. By that time, I was sufficiently blasé about flying as well as sufficiently tired that I stretched out on a soft-looking mail sack and slept most of the way. I blew into headquarters like a whirlwind, got Father on the phone to announce my arrival, and arranged a rendezvous for 2:30, which left me an hour and a half to while away as best I could.

Then Father was late, so in the best "Dr. Livingstone, I presume" style, I looked at my watch and chided him on his tardiness. I accompanied him while he tended to some business, and wrote my last letter while waiting for him. Then we went to his hotel and had a beginning of a real talk, then down to dinner, back to his room to talk some more and for him to try to give me almost everything he had:

I acquired two jigger-sized bottles of scotch; a beautiful woolen undershirt which he had bought in Bogota; *A Sense of Humus* which I already knew from its condensation in a magazine and which I was very glad to have in its entirety (finished now, and will go on to Richard); *Le Petit Prince* from you, Mother (I have started it and think it is one of the most completely charming books I have ever read. Many thanks); a can of Nescafé; four films for my camera, and last but not least, I borrowed some money so I could buy a new coat to take the place of my Red Cross one which was burned up when the dry cleaners had a fire. They promised to pay me fifty dollars for it, but the wheels had not gone around by the time I left, and my paycheck was somewhere en route, so I was almost penniless. I got the money, of course, and later got a WAC coat, not as heavy as the nurses' coats but better than none. Quite good looking and most useful.

In a "Dear Mother" letter later, I wrote:

I had the rest of the morning with Father (he promised me a hot bath at the hotel, but by the time my briefing was finished and I got there, the water was no longer hot). Then we had lunch together and I went to the airport with him, saying goodbye in a very casual fashion, thinking I would see him again in a few days. Maybe it was just as well that way.

Then I went to work. The rest of the week I worked hard all day and played quite hard most of the night. A few high spots come to mind. One was my walk down to work the first morning. I had been billeted in a very nice room *chez Mme Veuve Lopez*. Big double bed which she opened for me every night (the first night she had not met me at all as she was out when I arrived and I came back to go to bed long after she had retired. I had left my gaudy pajamas, just purchased at the PX, on the bed and my muddy field boots were in one corner. My suitcase was not unpacked. So all she saw was masculine, and the next morning when a sleepy girl said *"Bonjour, Madame"* she almost fell over in surprise. She had thought her new boarder was a man!) The apartment was way up on top of a hill, one could descend either by narrow streets or by steep flights of steps which led from one hairpin turn of the street to one at a higher level. It had rained in the night and temporarily everything was shining and clean. The sun had not been up very long and the sky was still tinged with pink. Lean and hungry cats were foraging in the trash cans on each corner. And chattering groups of pig-tailed, pinafored school children each one escorted by a prim and proper *bonne*, skipped down the streets, passed from time to time by an earnest bespectacled university student on his bicycle. Down on the main street, under the mulberry trees walked tidy housewives with long loaves of bread and baskets of vegetables and maybe a piece of ice wrapped up in paper. And Moslem women, modestly hidden behind their veils, hurried home on silent bare feet, perhaps from the mosque around the corner. To a little country girl like me it was really kind of fun seeing all the life and movement of a city.

The November 11 Armistice Day Parade was another high spot, even though it poured buckets during the whole thing. I missed part of it, but I hear that there was a detachment of Tuaregs on white camels, must have been quite something. They wore white burnooses with scarlet linings. There were many Goums, too, in brown almost habit-like tunics girdled at the waist, sandals on their bare feet and their shaved heads wrapped in brown turbans. Most of them little men with a cat-like softness to their walk. The WACs put on a fine show, marching better than anyone else, except the British groups. From all I hear, those girls are proving their worth and even the old diehards are admitting that they are pretty useful!

A comment in a bookstore may amuse you. Two very young sailors walked in, one of them remarking seriously to the other, "But even agnostics should go to see a beautiful cathedral!"

Then there was the delicious dinner I had with a French doctor and his family, in their luxurious apartment. They are one of the wealthiest families in town, owning a lot of property in town and vineyards and so forth around the countryside. We had an aperitif made from his own grapes, as was the wine we had at dinner, fresh-caught fish, lamb chops from his own farm, little sautéed squash, a wonderful green salad, an interesting cold pie made from corn meal and honey, sort of like an Indian pudding but in a pie crust, and finally very sweet mandarins from his own orange groves. It was quite a linguistic evening with French, Italian, Spanish and German, as well as English all being spoken (but not all very well). It was just a family gathering with the doctor and his wife, a son, a daughter and her husband and their beautiful eight-year-old boy, a child with big brown eyes and very blond hair, and charming manners. Far from a sissy, there was an impish twinkle in his eyes, particularly when his bedtime came, but he was quiet and very well behaved with the grownups, not in a restrained way, just a gentlemanly way, if you know what I mean.

Then there was the unbelievable afternoon when I first went to a hairdresser, had my hair washed and set, and then went back to the apartment and had a *hot bath in a bathtub!* (After first risking my life by lighting one of those infernal gadgets the French have for heating water. You know, a gas contraption. First you turn on the gas in the bathroom, then turn on the faucet and with a terrific roar and sometimes an explosion the gas burner lights and theoretically hot water pours immediately into the bathtub.) It was my first bath like that in eight months, (I told Madame that it was my first bath in that long and she sort of backed away from me until I explained we had cold showers!) I must admit I was a little disappointed. Maybe the water wasn't hot enough, or I wanted bath salts, or else that it was just so strange that I couldn't really enjoy it, but it did not live up to my expectations. Then I had a bit of the scotch that Father had given me and went out for dinner with Russ Dorr [son of special friends of the family] whom I had bumped into most unexpectedly. It was fun seeing him again, and we had a very pleasant evening.

But one of the most glamorous of all evenings was the one that I spent on board ship. Remind me to join the Navy in the next war, they really know how to live. The party started out as one of these wholesale invitation things; you know, a blanket invitation for a dozen girls for a dinner and dance. It was a cold, rainy and windy night. We walked along the beach for a little, watching the waves break and the rain slant down over the water. After signaling out to the ship, a landing barge was sent in for us, but the water was too rough for it to come right up on the beach. So some of the sailors hastily took off their shoes and rolled up their pants and carried us one by one out through the water to the barge. The squeals of some of the French girls with us made it sound all the more exciting. And we had to hurry as those barges cannot stay inshore more than a few minutes or they get grounded. Then out through the waves, with the moon just coming out from behind the rain clouds, to the ship, up a very long and steep companionway or whatever they are called, and into a *heated* room. The first heat like that since I left the States! We were really uncomfortably warm. I was paired off with a very nice boy from New Jersey, who later proudly yet rather shyly showed me a picture of his rather new wife. (I would love to have even one penny for each picture I've looked at and exclaimed over, since I got here! Thousands, I'm sure.)

The dining room was decorated with big red balloons, the tablecloths were white, we had napkins, and even a variety of forks and spoons so I had to keep a watchful eye on my escort to see which to use when! Dinner was of course delicious. Soup, chicken, fried potatoes, a vegetable, a fresh tomato and lettuce salad, real butter (I've had it a number of times since, but that was really the first in months and months. Wonderful.) They had four musicians from the show "Hey Rookie" play during dinner, coming around to each table to play requests. And then there was dancing and later ice cream and cake. And then home again in the barge, this time we had to get ourselves through the edge of the water, watching the waves and trying to run in between. Golly, what a grand evening, and sort of story-bookish.

There is lots more to tell you, but I guess I had better wait until my next letter. This one has acquired gargantuan proportions.

All that was written on November 24, after I got back to the 26th General which by then was set up in very temporary quarters outside Bizerte. Father had been delayed in Cairo where he had gone to meet with the consul general, Alex Kirk, with whom I had lunch a year later when he was our ambassador in Rome. So I wasn't able to see Father again as we'd planned after all. (Among my most precious papers is a long letter he wrote to Mother about our time together in Algiers and his stay in Cairo.) In my journal, I wrote briefly about a wonderful Cook's tour of Algiers one Sunday, visiting a mosque and even up and through the Casbah with a guide who had a vividly dramatic way of describing the places we visited.

It was with almost a sense of relief that I was recalled on Wednesday, November 17, to my unit. The personnel work was interesting and fun but tiring as I was so completely on my own and was often uncertain about the unilateral decisions I had to make. As usual, my scheduled departure was one of those "hurry up and wait" events . . . two hours at Maison Blanche (the airport for Algiers) but all flights canceled. So back to town, dinner at the Cercle Interallié where, according to my journal entry of November 18, General Giraud's brother joined us for cocktails. (General Henri Giraud succeeded Admiral François Darlan as the senior administrative official in French North Africa after the Vichy admiral was assassinated in December.) Later in the evening, I had to pay for this "heady" experience by spending the night in a bed with no blankets as I hadn't been expected to return. Cold as that was, it was nothing compared to the next night in a tent at the 33rd General Hospital outside Bizerte when the temperature went down to freezing and, although I had three blankets on top of me, there was nothing between me and the bare canvas of the cot. All in all it was a miserable week as we waited for embarkation orders. It was cold and rainy most of the time and Buff and I did little but sit around and chat with the nurses, knit, read, write letters and eat, either in the mess, or once at the French Naval Club in Ferryville.

My journal entry for November 28:

Got up at 5:15, loaded the ship at 8, sailed at 11. Gene

Spencer came down to see me off. Exciting and strange to be leaving Africa at last. Down past Cap Bon and Kelibia, Pantellaria about 8 P.M.: the end of my African adventure. It's been pretty grand and I wouldn't have missed it for anything. Our ship is a British hospital ship, the HMHS *Vasna*, a former P&O boat. The food is pretty good. We sleep 2 deep in crib-like bunks in one of the wards. Good to be out of the mud. Strange being on a lighted ship without a convoy.

The next day was beautifully sunny with calm blue waters, a real winter's Mediterranean cruise with snow-capped Mt. Etna in view most of the time. It was for us (just the nurse and Red Cross staff) a lovely two-day trip and very restful. But, for the majority of the officers and enlisted men who crossed on a Royal Navy LCI [Landing Craft Infantry], it was quite another story, one that lasted three and a half days. There were no bunks, very limited floor space and only long wooden benches divided into individual seats by metal arms. Below decks, diesel fumes and the hard wooden benches made the men miserable, while those who sought fresh air on deck were exposed to rain and ocean spray. On top of that, very rough stormy weather made even the sailors seasick. The LCI reached Taranto in Southern Italy on November 25, Thanksgiving Day, and as one passenger wrote, "we were sure that nowhere in the world was there a group of men more thankful!"

A third contingent of one officer and nineteen enlisted men from our hospital proceeded aboard the Liberty ship *Samuel J. Tilden* from Bizerte to our assigned location in Bari, Italy, an ancient seaport on the west coast of the Adriatic where St. Nicholas is reputedly buried. The vessel was big in comparison with the LCI, and the voyage itself was relatively uneventful. However, she arrived in the harbor of Bari just in time for an air raid in which the ship received a direct hit. The men were rescued but the ship sank with all the hospital equipment on board and most of our personal belongings, and this raid had awful consequences.

CHAPTER THREE

Italian Interlude

—◆—

November 30, 1943–March 22, 1944

The Luftwaffe bombing of Allied ships in the harbor of Bari, Italy, on December 2 was the most disastrous single air attack on Allied shipping since Pearl Harbor. It reminded us, as President Roosevelt said in his Christmas message, "There is no easy road to victory. And the end is not yet in sight."

Allied forces landed at Anzio, just north of Rome, in January and that same month the 900-day siege of Leningrad came to an end.

At home, the war effort would soon reach its peak, setting records for the production of war matériel of all kinds, including the C-47 transport plane and the Jeep. The nation was preparing for two amphibious invasions on opposite sides of the world.

The acronym SNAFU (for "situation normal, all fouled up") originated during World War II, and it certainly described our arrival in Taranto on November 30. I wrote in my journal:

Dropped anchor at eleven, almost two days to the hour. Then we sat and sat, ready to leave at a moment's notice. Then a British major came out in a boat and announced that we were not expected, no one knew we were there, there was no way of letting the hospital know we had come! So we may have to stay in some ward tents on a hill with a stove and our 50 cases of C rations! Lovely prospect . . . so we unpacked again and settled in for the afternoon. Then they said we would get off in the evening. So we hastily packed again. Then they said we could have tea first, but just as we got bread and jam, they called us to get off at once. So we pushed the bread into our mouths, grabbed our things and got into an LCM [Landing Craft Mechanized, designed to carry trucks and armored vehicles] singing as we pulled away from the ship.

A two-and-a-half hour ride in vehicles called weapons carriers brought us to Bari and the imposing stone and stucco buildings of the Ospedale Militare Lorenzo Bonomo just outside the city on the Corso Sicilia. *The History of the 26th General Hospital* described the setup:

The main buildings were placed one behind another, facing Corso Sicilia, and were connected by an enclosed stone and glass paneled corridor. . . . Along each side of the main building was a paved roadway, one lined with palms, the other with oleanders. There were other trees in the gardens and many varieties of shrubs and flowers. There were neatly trimmed hedges around the gardens and along some of the walks. Flowers were still in bloom and the whole picture was in marked contrast to our drab tent hospital in Africa.

It was dark by the time our convoy of nurses and Red Cross staff arrived from Taranto, and we were too tired to appreciate the beauty and convenience of our new hospital. All that really mattered at that point was something quick to eat and then to bed. Even the fact that bed was a canvas cot with only one blanket didn't matter too much; we had arrived and there was a roof over our heads. My first letter home was headed "Somewhere in Italy." My journal read:

Looks pretty good as far as work is concerned but living

74

won't be as much fun. Ten of us are in the Annex, five nurses in one room, four Red Cross in another, and Anne Aldridge in the front room. Small bathroom with just a WC and wash basin. Housekeeping instincts are all to the fore. Curtains and bedspreads came out of bedrolls, boxes are swiped on all sides. The Italians living in our basement are hired to wash the floors in return for some of our supper. Reminds me of the first day at college. Great exploring of the grounds and buildings. Lovely little chapel.

I "did the town" the next day, December 2, going in on the mail truck with a number of the doctors. We shopped for furniture most of the morning, buying chairs, coatracks and a mirror and ordering some big wardrobes. Prices seemed very reasonable and the quality quite good. The Annex was very appreciative of my purchases when I got back after supper in, of all novel experiences, a taxi.

However, I wasn't back half an hour before we heard the rumble of antiaircraft fire. Then came the thunderous bursts of big guns and the hospital lights went out. We put on our helmets and went up on the roof to watch the tracer bullets, flares and searchlights. As we were a few miles outside the city, we were in little actual danger although the shrapnel fell like hail around us. One tremendous explosion almost knocked us over so we retreated, wisely, to take shelter in our windowless hallway. After a period of almost ten minutes without any noise, I decided to venture into our bedroom to get my flashlight. The room was dark except for a brilliant orange glow beyond the closed shutters and I went over to the window to investigate. Just at that moment, the ammunition ship in the harbor exploded and the blast blew the window open in my face! Fortunately, it was loosely latched. Otherwise, the glass would have shattered and I probably would have been very badly cut. I moved faster than I ever had before and have no recollection of getting across the room and back into the safety of the hallway, having quite forgotten to bring my flashlight with me.

The results of the raid were very serious as all our hospital supplies were on the *Samuel J. Tilden* which was just entering the harbor when the enemy bombers attacked. Two direct bomb hits set fire to the ship and a British torpedo boat had to sink it later that evening. Miraculously all but one of the twenty-two 26th General Hospital personnel on board escaped, although some suffered very serious injuries. So at a time when hospital care was critically needed in the area, our hospital was almost completely without supplies and was further handicapped by the shortage of medical staff, causing a considerable delay in our being able to receive patients.

According to one account, there were seventeen ships sunk by Luftwaffe bombers and eight damaged, with 1,644 casualties among the Allied personnel, including 422 deaths. It was the most disastrous single air strike since Pearl Harbor. But the true horror of the night came when one of the damaged ships exploded—one of *our* ships, which was carrying chemical warfare agents including one hundred tons of mustard gas bombs that released poison over a wide area. Fuel oil spilled by the ships spread over the water and absorbed the toxic mustard gas, compounding the catastrophe. The definitive account[†] describes it thus:

> The men struggling in the harbor water, the civilians enveloped in the deadly clouds of smoke, and the rescuers working on the docks were all unaware of the presence of the gas and some died still not knowing about it. Others were blinded or burned. Hospital personnel treated the survivors for shock and exposure, not realizing they had been subjected to a chemical agent. It wasn't until many of the patients died

† Glenn B. Infield, *Disaster at Bari* (Macmillan 1971) 9-10.

without obvious causes that an investigation was launched and the true reason for the deaths learned.

The fact that the mustard gas was on one of our ships was, as Glenn Infield wrote, "one of the best kept secrets of World War II." His book is a truly horrifying account of what happened, based largely on personal accounts from people who were there, and includes a number of pages about the 26th General Hospital. My own account, taken from my journal, also reflects the horror.

Ours was the only American general hospital in Italy. We were able to set up an emergency hospital to operate on a limited basis when some supplies and equipment were obtained from Italian and other sources. Most of the casualties were taken to the British and New Zealand hospitals which were already in full operation nearby. Some of our medical staff were sent to assist in the hospitals, and the Red Cross was asked to assist in searching for missing American personnel, a task which extended as far as Brindisi and Taranto. I took part in this search. As I wrote later,

To add to the confusion and difficulties, while patients were being admitted to the British hospital, one of their walls collapsed from the blast and they had to move their own patients while they were admitting new ones. As you can imagine, this resulted in complete chaos as far as records were concerned and it was weeks before they had patients straightened out and identified. Many of course were unconscious as they were brought in and one of the jobs that fell to the Red Cross was the identifying of the hundreds of wounded. There were not nearly enough beds to go around and the litters were placed on the floors of lobbies and corridors. There were serious shortages of medical supplies and medicines. There was perhaps one thermometer for three hundred men. The nurses and doctors worked twenty hours or more a day, the nurses from our hospital coming down to help and relieve whenever possible. The whole scene reminded me of pictures of Florence Nightingale during the Crimean War. There wasn't even time to take out boys who had died—the blankets were pulled over their faces and I stepped over them to get to the living beyond. No outsiders except the nurses who had volunteered and the Red Cross workers were allowed in the hospitals and those of us in the Red Cross were the only source of information for almost a week as to the names and outfits of the casualties. Majors and colonels, commanding officers of nearby units, waited for us on the doorstep to find out if we had located missing men, and the War Shipping Board was so impressed by the work that one of my colleagues did that they tried to get her permanently assigned to their organization. Sometimes it would take us three hours to get a boy's complete name and unit. Patient questioning would bring out perhaps his first name before he slipped back into unconsciousness and we would have to wait until he came to again before we could get the rest of it. It was an unbelievable nightmare and an experience that I will never forget.

Because they were written as events occurred, my journal entries were even more graphic:

December 4: Went to the [British] 98th General Hospital today to help take care of the many American boys there from the Bari blitz. Even some of our own. The only way we could do it was to close our minds completely, smile and chat with the boys just as if they weren't burned to a crisp, blown to pieces and probably dying.

December 6: A very busy and tiring afternoon at the 98th. One doesn't dare even think there or it would make you sick. Buff and I had to step over a boy who had died and was lying on a stretcher, in order to get downstairs. The smells and sights and sounds remind me of the Coconut Grove fire in Boston just about a year ago.

December 10: Hospital getting more organized. Some of

our nurses on D.S. [detached service] at the 96th which helps a lot. But still a lot of very sick boys, several dying every day. One of our psychiatrists, Charlie Polan, made rounds with me today and even he was a bit taken aback by the conditions and the state of the patients. Mustard gas burns are not pretty.

After the mustard gas crisis passed, life became closer to normal, and there was even time to relax. My journal goes on to tell of many evenings with friends in a little cafe in a nearby village, a place we frequented so often that I later wrote an essay about "Mike's Place."

One of the most intriguing things about Italy is the number of people who speak English. Every little town seems to have at least one person in it who has lived in America for a number of years and who has come home with fabulous tales of the way the Americans behave, live and eat. When we drive through a tiny village and stop for directions, as likely as not someone will step up to the car and ask "Where you wanta go?" Or, as happened one day, a weary voice was heard over the babble of a small crowd which had sprung up from nowhere for no particular reason (as Italian crowds are wont to do) remarking earnestly "I wish to hell I was back in Chicago."

One such ex-American, in a small town not far from us, had returned home to open a barber shop. I think he got homesick for the United States from time to time, and welcomed any American customers, talking incessantly all the time he was shaving them or cutting their hair. The conversation turned to food, as it always does at one point or another, and the usual complaints of Vienna sausage, Spam and other G.I. delicacies were made. So the barber, eager to win the goodwill of his customer and also eager to bring a little of the taken-for-granted American wealth to his town and particularly to his friends, introduced us to Mike.

Mike was in peacetime, I think, the middleman between

the farmers of the region and the markets. At least that was the trade written on the card he gave us. But by inclination he was a bootlegger, barkeeper, a dealer in black market goods, and a lover of intrigue. He was a big fellow, not particularly tall but heavily built, and the war had not made him tighten his belt very much. He looked well fed and only his clothes kept him from looking prosperous. His dark suit was rather shabby and the sweater under his coat far from clean. I never saw Mike without his hat, which sometimes he wore forward on his head in a sinister fashion and sometimes pushed way back in moments of stress and excitement, so he could get at his forehead to wipe it off with a dirty handkerchief or slap with the flat of his hand to express extreme emotion.

The street in front of Mike's Place was narrow and dirty and muddy. You pushed open a little door in a wall and stepped into a courtyard which was also very muddy and which had a little outhouse built into the wall on the left. At the far end of the courtyard was the door of the house, so low that even I had to stoop a bit to go in, and in front of the door itself hung one of those strange curtains made of wooden beads on long strings. The public bar is in the front room, and usually the air is blue with smoke and heavy with the sweet smell of the *"vino nero"* that is so good here. Very few American soldiers come to this bar, but the British and New Zealanders crowd the place every night.

The conversation and snatches of song stop for a moment as we make our way through the room. A few boys say good evening to us, a few half stand up seeing an officer and a girl, but as soon as we are through the door into the back part or the house, their momentary curiosity and interest are forgotten and they are back into their own worlds again. Through a low archway and up a few steps and we are in our own private world too. It is a sort of a dining room, but I think the family use it very seldom, preferring the warmth of the kitchen which is through another even smaller door and down five or six very steep steps to the right. The only furniture in this room is a rather elegant cupboard with glass doors on the top half, a big heavy wooden table, seven or eight chairs of varying designs and sizes, and a large not too soft horsehair sofa which is used for a great many things. We sit on it when we are there; the dog keeps one of his bones pushed down behind the cushion; two of the children are often tucked onto it, well wrapped in shawls and coats, to sleep until the family retires upstairs; coats are piled on it; dishes are set on it—in fact it is a very useful piece of furniture. The room is separated from the back hall and the side stone steps that lead upstairs by a partition that reaches halfway to the ceiling, with a window and door cut in it making the room nice and breezy on cold winter nights. The breeze and the cold stone floor give a sort of refrigerator chill to the place and make warm clothes essential.

As we come in, Mike's wife comes up the steps from her kitchen to greet us with a smile and a *"Buona sera."* She is chubby and plump, and, still pretty—was probably a real beauty when she was younger. Her brown hair, now a little faded, is piled in a knot on top of her head and her pleasant round face is dominated by her dark brown eyes. She takes Mike and his emotional storms and his guests and his problems very calmly, having known him so long she can no longer get excited every time he does. The children, shy at first, soon get to know us and run to greet us when we come in, hoping for candy or a piece of chewing gum. There is dark little Melina who is a round butterball of a child and already looks like her mother, and then there is the very blond, almost Germanic looking little child Michele, Mike Junior, who doesn't look one bit like his father. Melina is a good, placid child and very affectionate as soon as she has accepted you as a friend, but Michele has his father's temperament if not his looks. Michele must be the center of the stage and he doesn't care if he gets his attention by being naughty or by smiling winningly at you. One time he will pull the dog's tail, or whisper naughty words in Melina's ear, causing her to break into tears and the next time he will sit like the little angel he resembles.

My favorite is the baby, who doesn't belong to Mike at all. Philomena is the daughter of an Italian sergeant who is in Sicily now, they think. She is about two months old and is one of the most friendly and social babies I have ever known. Her mother is probably a younger sister of Mike's wife, but I've never been able to quite figure that relationship out. She is as charming as Philomena is, being slim and dark, with big black eyes and long hair braided in a coronet around her head. She very willingly turns Philomena over to me when I come in, probably glad to be able to forget her daughter for even half an hour. The baby is usually wrapped in swaddling clothes, which are bound almost up to her armpits and which give practically the feeling of a plaster cast on her legs and body. It is so stiff that they can stand the baby up in a corner just as one would a package. Once, however, she was without her wrappings and I was relieved to see that she had little pink toes and curling feet, just like other babies.

There are others in the family, and many friends who wander in and out. The ramifications of an Italian family are quite complicated, I imagine, and the only other person we have been able to identify is Mike's mother, who obviously runs the place, Mike, the children and anyone who comes within the scope of her reaching voice. Mike may be able to yell for his wife or his cousin or his sister, but he subsides whenever his mother is around, and then she yells for him. Italians seem to be always yelling. The nearer they are to you, the more noise they make. And what seems to be a terrific fight with severe injury if not immediate death threatening the two most active participants, will turn out to be a discussion of the weather or an inquiry as to the baby's health.

The food is the chief reason for our frequent visits to Mike's Place. Bring him a little white flour, a little sugar, perhaps a chicken or maybe not even that, and you will get a meal fit for the gods and Italians. The best tablecloth is brought out of the cupboard and spread lovingly on the table. Places are set for us and decanters of both red and black wine brought in. Two large earthenware dishes, like giant pie plates and filled with hot coals and ashes, are put under the table. It is amazing how much heat these give out, and they make all the difference in the world. If one's feet are warm the rest of one seems to be warm too, or a reasonable facsimile of same. During the evening they have to be stirred up once or twice (the coals, not one's feet).

The first course is, of course, antipasto. There are always pickled strips of green pepper and little anchovies in olive oil. But sometimes as a special treat, there are wonderful bits of artichoke hearts, also in olive oil. The best way to eat is to alternate the antipasto with sips of wine, using the dark bread to push with and then later to soak up the leftover olive oil, which is delicately flavored with the anchovies and artichokes and the spices used on these. After the antipasto we sometimes have a soup, a warm filling cabbage soup or a clear soup with noodles on the nights we have turkey. Then comes one of the *spécialitiés de la maison,* shell noodles with cheese and tomato sauce. The first time I had this I thought it might be the main course, and ate accordingly, much to my later grief. The plates are piled high with the steaming shells, and you soon learn that you cannot eat fast enough to keep up with your enjoyment if you use a fork. So forks are discarded and spoons taken up. These plates, empty against one's better judgment, are taken away, and the *pièce de résistance* is brought on.

This varies according to what we have brought them the day before or what we have ordered. Once it was steak with french fried potatoes; once it was turkey cacciatore. Once it was two kinds of fish which we had asked Mike to buy for us, one a bony sort of sea bass, and one an eel steak; and once, on New Year's night, when we were full of food and drink and too much party, they seemed to know just what we wanted and without asking brought us two fluffy omelettes. With eggs as scarce over here as they are, that was a real treat and just what our jaded appetites wanted.

During this part of the meal there is usually not a great deal of conversation. The food is too good to be spoiled by a lot of talking. Mike is busy out in the bar, so his mother, his wife and the rest of the family are down in the kitchen, the children are getting sleepy and quieter, and we are eating. From time to time there is a loud series of knocks on the back door, reminiscent of speakeasy days, and one of the family will hurry to answer it, opening the door just a crack to see who is there. But as the bar is still officially open, most of the backdoor business consists of friends of the family who are coming to spend an evening with them, or patrons of the "pension" they run upstairs, not a very high class one, I would judge, from the looks of the people on their way up. Later, however, when we have reached the dessert or even the liqueur stage, the backdoor clientele is of a different sort. The MPs have closed the bar and made everyone leave by the front door. Then they and their friends return, by the back door, for another hour or so of quiet drinking. Occasionally some undesirables find this back door and there is much voluble arguing in two languages.

Mike is usually hesitant about calling the MPs to his help and will even bring a drink to someone in the back hall in preference to getting assistance in ejecting them. One night when there were no MPs around, and two New Zealand soldiers were insistent about coming in, the two officers with me, being Welshmen, could no longer restrain their curiosity and their desire to be in the thick of things. So they joined the argument by the back door. Mike and the Colonel, backed with the imposing height of the Lieutenant, had just persuaded the men to leave and come back the next day and the Colonel had just stooped to pick up a cap which had been dropped, when a whirlwind hit him from behind, lifted him off the floor and propelled him some fifteen feet through the door and into the back alley. Mike's wife, becoming worried and fearing it could turn into a real fracas, had enlisted the help of a young and wiry *Fascista* cousin. He had come in from the front room, saw a group by the door but had no way of knowing which was friend and which was foe. So he just picked on someone he knew did not belong to his family and pushed him out. The tall Lieutenant turned on him with rage, and shook him, much as a big dog would shake a rat. But everyone soon realized what had happened, the Colonel was brought in out of the night, none the worse for his sudden trip. The young Fascist apologized in Italian and kissed the Colonel's hand in an excess of abashment, glasses were filled and everybody's health was toasted. For the rest of the evening and in fact every time after that, nothing was too good for us. Mike even brought out an extra special table wine, reminiscent of an excellent cider.

By the time we have reached dessert, we are no longer quite as hungry as when we arrived and we are grateful that the meal doesn't include a heavy sweet to end with. Usually there are oranges and walnuts and figs stuffed with almonds, but sometimes a few stalks of fennel, or *finocchio* as it is called in Italy, are added as an extra delicacy. The only time we had a sweet to eat when we had brought them flour and sugared cocoa and they made us, as a special treat, the cake of cakes. It had thick white frosting on it, decorated with bits of citron and maraschino cherries, and inside was custard fill-ing, both plain and chocolate, and almonds, and cake and who knows what else. It was incredible, a veritable master-piece. I got pleasure eating it, but am sure that Mike's wife got even more pleasure out of making it. It must have been a long time since she had had all the necessary ingredients, and the citron had probably been stored away waiting for some special occasion.

The only times that we have coffee are when we bring it to them. Once we had a regular demitasse, and once we had a delectable mixture of coffee and cocoa, thick like Turkish coffee and tasting something like bitter chocolate as the coffee took most of the sweetness from the cocoa. Always we have a liqueur, a home product. Sometimes it is a cloudy sort of lemony liqueur and sometimes it tastes a little like anisette, but it is always good. Then cigarettes come out, chairs are pushed back a bit, and about this time Mike drops in for a chat, if it can be called that with his Italian and our English. One never-to-be-forgotten evening he was followed in by a little disheveled, rat-faced individual who sort of slunk up the stair after him. We paid no attention to him and continued making comments in English *sotte voce* about our attempts to talk with Mike. Suddenly Rat-face spoke "Excuse me, but have you got a match?" We almost fell over, and hastily cast back our thoughts pondering what we had said that could have been heard.

Like so many others, he had lived in the States for years. He became an unwilling interpreter for the rest of the evening, explaining Mike's political tirades to us and our responses to Mike. Mike was very pro-American that evening, and couldn't understand why the Americans, Mr. Roosevelt especially, couldn't take Italy over as a sort of colony and run it for them. He wanted us all to live in Italy after the war, and lots of Italians to go to America. He became more and more excited, and one after the other the rest of the family drifted in, forming an admiring circle for Papa's histrionics. If you had seen it in the movies, your first feeling would have been that it was overdone, that it was a bit of overacting, but it really was happening and we had a difficult time controlling our laughter.

Finally the foot warmers burn down, finally we notice that the room has become quite chilly, finally we notice that we have been there about three hours, and we make our departure. We must sign the ration book for bread, and we must pay the ridiculously small bill for our dinner with no charge for the warmth, the service, the entertainment and the goodwill. The whole family follows us to the door and bows us out. The street is dark and quiet, the night is frosty cold, the stars are incredibly bright and the church clock chimes out the quarter hour.

During my Italian interlude, even work could be fun. From time to time, I had the enviable assignment of escorting ambulatory patients to the opera or symphony. It was a *Through the Looking Glass* experience to sit in the Royal Box in a real theater listening to Beethoven's Fifth or watching Verdi's *La Traviata*, especially as on the way we often passed streams of refugees fleeing the city. The roads were often crowded with people and wagons piled high with all their belongings and those too young or too old to walk. Some had horses to pull the carts, others were pulled by the men.

My letters home were intentionally less detailed about the really traumatic experiences. On December 19, I glossed over what I had been doing with a simple sentence about how busy we were visiting American patients in a British hospital in addition to our own work. I went on to describe my own pleasant living conditions and social life, which centered around the sitting room we had made out of the windowless hall and where we had carol sings and guessing games by candlelight. I had bought a Christmas tree that we set up in the hall and we enlisted all visitors into our decoration-making endeavors: stringing Life Savers on red yarn, punching holes in Necco wafers and hanging them, and making balls and icicles from the cellophane wrappings on cigarette packages. I wrote:

The boys loved it and when the electricity is on we use our hot plate and make coffee, tea or bouillon to order . . . The fellows come early for their dates with other girls so that they can spend half an hour with us first. One of the doctors calls them "the termites," they are underfoot so constantly . . . at times it is something of a nuisance but they get so much

87

pleasure out of it and that, too, is part of our Red Cross work —though we would never tell them so.

My letter ended with requests for replacements of various items, including shoes which had been on the ill-fated ship carrying all our supplies and most of our personal belongings. I concluded, "It doesn't seem right that *any* enjoyment should come out of anything so terrible. I wish I could do something harder and more demanding and more contributory to the war effort." So I articulated the first stirrings of restlessness, feelings which would eventually lead me to leave the Red Cross. Christmas Eve I had supper on board a very small ship which was engaged in ferrying refugees, Americans, British, Partisans and Chetniks [Yugoslav resistance people] across the Adriatic to and from Yugoslavia. For security reasons, I referred to my English date as an "alphabetic stepbrother or something." My guess fifty years later is that I meant to indicate he was with British intelligence. I commented in my journal that the supper was a meager meatless one as most of the group was going to midnight Mass, but the conversation was fascinating and stimulated my interest in the Balkans, an interest which I nurtured by reading Rebecca West's *Black Lamb and Grey Falcon*, Louis Adamic's *My Native Land*, and Michael Padev's *Escape from the Balkans*. I got to know the people in Bari who were involved in intelligence work and in early January began to make some serious inquiries about other employment. My letters home had to be very vague about the whole thing for security reasons, but as I had talked with Father about it when we were together in Algiers, I could refer indirectly to these activities.

In between everything else, I fell in love again! "Dear John" letters are traditionally written from the girl at home to the guy overseas, but in my case it was the girl overseas who wrote to the guy at home. It was not an easy letter that

I wrote while still in North Africa, having slowly come to the conclusion that we really had little in common. If he had been overseas too it might have turned out differently; as it was I felt my experiences were so completely different from his that they created a gap in our relationship that would be difficult if not impossible to bridge after the war. I was, therefore, relatively fancy-free when I met Doug, my new beau. We shared many activities, including frequent meals at "Mike's Place" during my remaining months in Bari and my letters home were full of references to him, places we'd gone and things we'd enjoyed together. (No, dear reader, that didn't survive the war either, but it was very special while it lasted.)

Between my professional activities and my social life, my letters home were a bit skimpy, but I made up for my temporary neglect with a long letter on January 16, part of which follows:

Here we go again. I'm going to try and remember back as far as Boxing Day, (the day after Christmas, in case you have forgotten), but I haven't my diary here, only my little engagement book and I don't know how good my memory is this morning.

Boxing Day we celebrated with Jimmie, Dickie and Red, three British boys we have sort of adopted. The whole week of Christmas and New Year's they were on leave, and they practically lived with us, coming over in the morning for no good reason, dropping in for tea and staying past supper time, coming in the evening to drink a little wine and maybe sing a bit. They're nice boys but completely crazy and a bit wearing after a while. But their Boxing Day party was one of the best I've been to. Most British parties are sort of catch-as-catch-can affairs but this one was different. The boys did nothing but devote themselves to giving us a good time. There was scotch to drink, delicious turkey, and other kinds of sandwiches, nuts and oranges and cookies and cakes, and even ice cream and coffee, the music was very good and they interspersed the regular dancing with things like the Polly Glide, the Lambeth Walk, and others. They introduced us to everyone, saw that we always had a partner, plied us with food and drink until I thought I would bust, and even saw to it that I won a prize for the "Spot Dance." The prize was a pair of silk stockings and a rather charming little doll in a lovely big box with designs on it. The doll is really just a head coming out of a lot of fluffy skirt, and is, I think, a *Lenci* [a popular brand] or an imitation. It is really rather sweet—I'll try and get it in the mails this week, Joan, as a present for you. You can put it on your bed at school or something, or don't people do that any more?. . .

New Year's Eve was a big brawl in one of the hotels, a super deluxe Cecil B. de Mille affair with delicacies that had been flown in from somewhere, two orchestras taking turns so the music never stopped, very bad liquor and too many "wolves." I went with Charlie Polan but might just as well have gone by myself for all I saw of him. Not that it was his fault. The high spot of the evening came when I acquired a canary. Apparently, they had a big pie with a bird cage on top (this is all hearsay, I didn't see any of it) and they opened the cage, letting all the birds out, and then cut the pie. A slightly inebriated Englishman came up to me with a canary in his hand, saying that he couldn't make the b——— bird stay in the tree (a potted palm in the lobby). So I rescued the little thing and found a small box for him and took him home with me. He seemed all right the next morning and I fed him a piece of dry bread and gave him some water, but when I got home at lunchtime, he had died. From fright, probably.

New Year's Day I was one of six girls asked to be sort of hostesses at an eggnog party for some personages of considerable rank. It was a lovely wild and windy day, and what I wanted to do most was to take a walk in the country or on the beach or something, but what with the eggnog party and then the cocktail party here at the hospital and then New Year's Dinner, I wasn't able to. That was the night Doug and I went to Mike's and had a delicious omelette and then came right home at the unheard-of early hour of nine o'clock.

My first real day off came last Thursday. I went into town right after breakfast planning to spend the whole day just walking around and exploring. I even took my flashlight so I could stay in for supper if I wanted to. I had the morning to myself and did just what my fancy dictated, first walking along the waterfront, watching the early morning sun on the little waves, the fishing boats riding gently at anchor, the nets spread out on the walks to dry, with one fellow sitting cross-legged in the middle of a net, skillfully mending a big hole. A little way out a rowboat was bobbing up and down, making its way to the quay. The oars were the biggest and heaviest I have ever seen and the rower had to cross them in front of himself in order to row. He was singing lustily as he rowed and the mender of nets was humming the same tune softly as he worked. The sky was blue, the sun warm, the water sparkling—and the war seemed very far away.

The next hour or so I just walked, first up one street and then down another. Then I found a little hat store and the temptation was too great. I went in and convulsed myself and everyone in the store by trying on silly little hats with veils—just the thing with a uniform. But even sillier, I bought two! They really are attractive and only cost $7 for the two of them, and it did bolster my morale (which is low these days).

I met one of our doctors about ten-thirty and we did some more shopping. He found a medical supply house and bought some things for his work, I bought a fairly good tennis racquet, and we browsed in several bookstores and I finally got a guidebook to Italy. Unfortunately, it is in Italian so I don't know how much good it will do me.

I have two little guidebooks to the town, which I found by happenchance, so after lunch we set out to explore the old part of town, not the modern (or at least more modern) shopping part. For two hours we wandered in and out of little narrow winding streets, under archways, past churches, into open squares you would never guess were there. From almost the first step, we lost our way on the map I had, so we contented ourselves with picking the narrowest and most devious alleys. We almost started a riot when we gave a couple of pieces of candy to three or four small children in one of the squares. From nowhere, hundreds of children appeared, pulling our coats, dragging at our hands and crying for candy.

We tried to pin down the difference between this town and some of the towns in North Africa which we had explored in a similar fashion. Both are dirty, very dirty, but somehow the dirt here seems cleaner. Looking through the narrow doorways, down the steps into a family's living room, there is much more of an attempt at comfort and cleanliness as we know it. There doesn't seem to be quite as much sickness and disease, the children are dirty but not covered with sores and flies and there is more of an attempt to clothe them sufficiently if not completely . . .

Did I ever tell you what a reputation Father has with us? When I got around to packing before leaving North Africa, I decided that four boxes of that flat toilet paper were more than I could pack, so I gave one box to Mary Mock, one to Buff and one to Fran. Later on, when we were staging, frequently there was no paper in the latrine first thing in the morning, so Buff would say as we started up the hill, "Wait a minute, let's get some of Mr. Phenix!" Apparently she had carried her box with her on the trip there, and the phrase "Some of Mr. Phenix's toilet paper" had soon become abbreviated to just "Mr. Phenix." So that is the stock expression. Everyone is most grateful to Mr. Phenix, and many of the nurses have enjoyed his present! But, used as I am to the phrase, it still makes me giggle when I hear it.

Various oblique references in my journal in January indi-

cated slow but encouraging progress toward a more interesting job. I saw some possible future colleagues a number
of times socially and my father was working on things
through channels in Washington and New York. I wrote
him a separate "business" letter on January 24 saying that I
was very pleased with his apparently favorable "progress
report." I commented how much I was enjoying "my recent
contacts both work and play, with some of the colleagues of
that chap 'F' had referred to me when I was tearing the
town apart for quick transportation to my family reunion. If
you follow me. It amuses me no end." (Translated, I was
referring to intelligence people to whom the consulate in
Tunis had introduced me when I was trying to get to
Algiers to meet Father on his way to Cairo.)

Then I went on, first to share with him the wonderful
concert I had attended in town and to apologize for "the
fall-off" of my correspondence home. I said that at first I
thought it was due to lack of time and energy but then realized that

more than ever before, many of the things I do or see or hear
are of such a nature that they cannot be told about yet. I suppose it is because one is closer to the scene of activity that
the censorship regulations are stricter. But I'm having an
awful time trying to remember all the things I want to tell
you after the war.

I hope I did remember to tell him some of them, but the
span of fifty years has taken its toll on my memory and I am
very frustrated by how much I have forgotten.

In February, my hospital duties were expanded to include
visiting American Field Service men hospitalized in a
nearby Allied hospital. As the AFS units were attached to
the British Army, the men were not eligible for treatment in
American hospitals which seemed to me then—and still

seems—unnecessarily bureaucratic. Some of them were very young and very homesick and very appreciative of my visits and the cigarettes, magazines and other things I brought them. One expressed his appreciation by taking me out to dinner and the theater when he was discharged. We ended the evening by having drinks in a British bar. As I wrote home, "The high point of the evening came when a young Canadian staggered over to me, said some very nice things about American girls, and then leaning over, asked seriously 'Would you mind if I called you Toots?' I hid my smiles and said it was perfectly all right." Today I would be expected to be offended, but in 1944 remarks like that were not considered "sexual harassment."

A V-mail letter to my father in February, written almost entirely in the third person about a "friend" who wanted to change jobs, ended with the comment, "Isn't this letter a masterpiece?" I was obviously getting more and more dissatisfied with the work I was doing (which some years later I unkindly described as helping take care of drunken airplane drivers), and more and more impatient with the necessary paperwork and red tape, much of which had to be done indirectly and through long-distance channels about my employment with another agency. Even so, many years later, I can feel the mood in which it was written and I think it must have delighted my father whose sense of official security was so ingrained.

A letter from Mother said Father advised no more packages, so things were apparently hotting up, and I replied by cable and then wrote on February 19 that I hoped the cable, with its approval of the "alternate plan," was comprehensible. My preoccupation with my own problems and uncertainties colored most of my journal entries and letters home. But there were, of course, some distractions: expeditions to explore the old town including the Church of St. Nicholas, and drives down to picturesque places like Alberobello and Castel del Monte, past olive groves and villages of *trulli* houses, those curious little whitewashed huts with straw beehive roofs. And frequent dinners at Mike's with Doug and/or others, trips to the opera, symphony or theater and even a masked Mardi Gras ball in late February.

March 1 was a red-letter day. My journal entry reads as follows:

At last the letter came. Washington has written [to the Red Cross in Algiers] re my resignation. I could die of excitement . . . Plan to leave the 15th. Met my friend "C" who has offered me a job with him and is crazy keen to send a signal on it to his boss, without my name, so he can reply to an inquiry with my name. I told him he was too late, that I was accepting a State Department appointment.

Another third-person letter on March 3 expressed our "mutual friend's" gratitude for all Father's advice and assistance and reassured him that as far as her Army associates were concerned, she was leaving the area and going to headquarters for reassignment. "The Red Cross associates understand she has been offered a State Department job but that a definite posting won't be done until after final clearance from the Red Cross."

I was excited but obviously more than a little apprehensive about leaving the security of my Red Cross identity, if only temporarily, for that of a plain civilian. And I felt very badly about leaving Buff and Fran—Mary Buffum (now Hamlin) and Frances Waterbury (now Richardson)—my two congenial Red Cross colleagues. However, I got my finances cleared up and requested travel orders to go to Algiers by way of Naples, and sent a radiogram to Red Cross national headquarters in Washington with a personal message to Father: "Resignation effective March 15th, leaving that date for Headquarters for release, reply."

And then, just to add to my feeling of insecurity, a letter from Father said everything had been called off because the job had already been filled due to numerous delays. The State Department got tired of waiting! Poor Father when he gets my message. And poor me. After talking with my friend 'C,' he came right over, again offering me a job, a place to stay, money, anything I might need. But I felt I had really burned my bridges and had best go ahead with my arrangement to go to Algiers. So I wrote Father on March 8:

Yesterday I felt quite like an orphan, sort of as though I had just jumped off a high cliff, thinking it only a few feet to the ground and then discovering the distance immeasurable. But my parachute is working nicely and I am now gently swimming in the air, adequately supported and slowly floating down to terra firma. Where I will land, I do not yet know, but that makes it all the more exciting. Hoping to hear from you soon, but for heaven's sake don't worry.

March 18 was the day of my departure and my journal reflects my ambivalent feelings, my regret about leaving my friends, my anxiety about the future and, in spite of everything, a joyful anticipation of new adventures and experiences. I flew to Naples on a medical evacuation plane over snowcapped mountains, dumped my unbelievable amount of baggage at the Red Cross office at the airfield, and was adopted by the Red Cross man there and a friendly lieutenant. They took me to lunch and then on an overnight trip to Ravello, driving over the same snow-capped mountains. I was so excited to see snowdrifts again that I got them to stop the car so I could get out and make snowballs! Down the lovely Salerno valley and along the coast to Ravello. Stayed in a *real* hotel with beds and sheets and rugs on the floor and even my own bathroom! Big dinner, drinks in front of an open fire and early to bed in spite of my escort's protests. It had been a long and wonderful day and I was tired.

I got up early the next morning and went to church in Assisi where St. Francis lived. Then down to Amalfi to do some shopping before the drive back to Naples. Ten minutes after I got back to the Red Cross office who should walk in, having learned of my arrival, but that special family friend, Alex de Bondini, who was stationed in Naples at that time as a sergeant in the American Army (because he was a naturalized citizen he was not eligible for officer training when he enlisted). He took me out to tea with some of his titled Italian friends who were living in Naples. It was highly amusing to see Alex in his American uniform with sergeant's stripes, bowing with great and obviously long-accustomed elegance over the hands of the various duchesses (and even a princess!) to whom he introduced me. I had left all my civilian clothes at the airport and in my rather travel-rumpled Red Cross uniform I wished I had some of his polished and graceful manners. We ended up having supper with some cousins in a little apartment right on the edge of a cliff overlooking the Bay of Naples with Vesuvius erupting on the horizon—the worst eruption since 1906. A very dramatic end to a fairy-tale day.

I did some inconclusive and unsatisfactory job hunting on Monday, somehow managed to miss my plane on Tuesday, and finally arrived in Algiers on Wednesday March 22 and cabled Father: "I HAVE LEFT HOSPITAL YOU ARE MORE THAN EVER IN MY THOUGHTS AT THIS TIME LOVE ELIZABETH"—meaning, of course, that my severance from the Red Cross was final and I was hoping for word from him via the Red Cross office in Algiers about a new job.

CHAPTER FOUR

Dark of the Moon
❖

March 22–July 9, 1944

Early in the spring, American B-17 Flying Fortresses penetrated deeper and deeper into Germany as they sought to destroy German industry and the Nazi war machine. Allied troops freed Rome on June 4 and two days later the landings in Normandy prepared the way for the liberation of France.

In the Pacific, U.S. Navy flyers heavily damaged Japanese naval aviation in the Philippines, and Saipan in the Marianas was captured by U.S. forces on July 9. From there the new B-29 bombers would now be able to reach Tokyo.

On June 22 the G.I. Bill of Rights was approved by Congress, enabling millions of war veterans to obtain funds for college education after the war.

Arriving in Algiers, I spent the next day filling out papers, talking to former employers and colleagues and prospective new ones, and arranging for a place to live. Some of the reasons for the delays and confusions were clarified weeks later when I received a wonderful long letter from my father. It was written on April 1 after his return from a trip to Washington where he had been able to talk to people in the State Department, Red Cross and Office of Strategic Services whose chief, General

99

"Wild Bill" Donovan, was a family friend. (I had gone to Potomac School, a private elementary school in Washington, with his daughter Patsy.) Apparently the original plan had been for me to go directly from Algiers to Madrid but the urgent need for a secretary in Algiers had persuaded the powers that be in Washington to assign me temporarily to the OSS office there, with the understanding that I would go on to Madrid later. So it was that after many weeks of indecision and uncertainty, with breathtaking speed my resignation from the Red Cross was accepted, and within 48 hours I started my new job with the Office of Strategic Services. I wrote home that I suspected much of the warmth and pleasure with which I was welcomed was due to the fact that I possessed my own typewriter, which "immediately put me in the same class as a chap who has access to two refrigerators!"

The "dark of the moon" is the last night or two of the moon's fourth quarter and the first night or two of the first quarter, when nights are darkest and provide cover for clandestine work—such as parachuting agents into Nazi-occupied France to link up with the French Underground. My letters barely refer to the activities that phrase implies—for security reasons, of course. First and foremost a secretary, I spent much of my time taking dictation and typing the memos, letters and cables that dealt with our unit's secret work, which centered on briefing the agents to be dropped into France and processing the information received from them and other agents elsewhere. Our agents had to be supplied with false identification papers, travel documents, ration cards, etc. as well as with clothes suitable for their "cover," and great care was taken that nothing—shoelaces, clothing labels, etc.—would betray their true identity. I was involved in all this almost daily, first in my office in an Army compound, later in a very pleasant villa farther out in the country which gave us more privacy and security. Several times I was allowed to go to the airfield during the dark of the moon. These were moments of deep emotion and high drama—the drive to the field, the waiting planes, the last-minute check of equipment, the clasp of hands as we bade farewell to men we had come to know while they had been with us. We always waited until the planes were out of sight before returning quietly to our billets.

My letters home were mostly about the delightful French family with whom I was billeted and about my various non-classified activities. Some letters were sent via regular APO [Army Post Office] airmail but some, when I was especially pressed for time, went V-mail—as "barely legible miniature letters photographed on microfilm and printed on slimy gray paper." They were hard enough to read fifty years ago; now I must use a magnifying glass in order to sort out the contents.

As I wrote home on March 25:

It is now 6:15 at the end of my first day at my new job, and I am slightly confused and befuddled by the variety of people, places and things I have come across. However, I am also very happy and think I will be much more content and occupied here than I was with the hospital. Whatever else I may lack, I am sure it will never be work.

The weather is lovely today, to celebrate my arrival perhaps, but I think the rainy season here is largely over and from now on we will have those heavenly days that I remembered with such nostalgia from last spring. I am fortunate in that I am not in the centre of town and that my billet with a French family is far enough away from town so that I have the feeling of being in the country, especially as there is a large and pretty garden all around the house. My room looks very comfortable, even has a little closet wash basin off it, and Madame has promised that I can have a hot bath twice a week and that she will serve me my *petit déjeuner* every morning. The bed looks soft, there is an easy chair by a small window, the furnishings are attractive, and all in all I expect to be very pleased with the setup. I hope that my linguistic abilities will be improved by the close association that way; the little Italian I learned only helped confuse me.

It was strange, but I had almost the sense of coming home when I arrived here the other day. I had never particularly liked the town before, but it is so much nicer than my last location that I am already quite fond of it. And it helps no end to be able to read signs and ask directions and talk to people with a reasonable facsimile of fluency.

The hours will probably be long here, both of necessity and because I will want to make them so. I have a feeling I will be loath even to take my day off. The people all seem most congenial and are very friendly and helpful.

Having inherited letter-writing genes from both sides of the family, the fact that I couldn't write about my job, except very indirectly, didn't discourage me from sending long "chatty" letters. The family with whom I was billeted were delightful people and I wrote in great detail about them.

April 1, 1944

Dear Mother and Father:

Lo and behold, a quiet few minutes at the end of the day. . . .

As I have told you, I am billeted with a very charming French family. There is M. and Mme. Andre, a daughter who is still in high school—she is 19, I think—and a son who is in the Army even though he doesn't seem much older. Mme. Andre works every day and I seldom see her. I think she must teach in some school, because she is home in the afternoons but she leaves before I come downstairs in the morning. M. Andre is delightful, he is always *en train* of shaving or dressing or weeding the garden or something. He and I quite frequently have *petit dejeuner* together—he does all the talking and I just smile and nod my head. My French at any time is not casually fluent, if I want to carry on a con-versation it cannot be the light just-tossed-off-remark sort of thing—and to have to make small talk in French at break-fast—well, it is just too much. But I am perfectly happy to sit and listen to M. Andre talk about one thing or another. I really understand almost all of it.

I usually wake up shortly before seven and luxuriously lie in bed, knowing that I don't have to get up for another half hour or so. I can look out my window and see the white pigeons preening themselves against the blue sky. The rooster in the yard below is most considerate and doesn't start his triumphant crowing until quite late in the early morning, there is a puppy in the next yard who whimpers a bit from time to time, and the pigeons coo softly to each other. Every morning so far has been sunny—I really think that there is nothing anywhere (except maybe Chocorua) like spring in North Africa.

About 7:20 there is a gentle thump outside my door and I know it is time to get up as my pitcher of hot water has just arrived.

Damn it, my boss has just arrived with an armful of work to be done. Duty calls—looks like this might be another late night and I was all set to go home right after supper (for the first time since I got here) and go to bed with a book. Nuts. However, I cannot complain, as I asked for it, didn't I? And I like it better this way, anyway. I went out last night, for my first real date since I got here, and all it did for me was to make me so lonesome for D[oug] that I could have wept, and did . . .

Sunday morning

I was right, there was a lot of work to do last night. . . . To go back to my "day." I reluctantly arise just before 7:30 and perform my ablutions in the little closet with a washbasin in it which adjoins my room, and wash out a pair of stockings or so, if the water is hot enough to be diluted down suffi-ciently. Mme. Andre took me downstairs one of my first mornings and showed me where the big wash tubs were and where the laundry lines were in the back yard, and I have a feeling that she disapproves of my hanging the stuff on hangers in my room, but it would take so much time and be so inconvenient to go through all that just for a few stockings. The rest of my stuff I can get washed elsewhere, I had forgotten how expensive laundry was in North Africa. Last week I paid 75 francs for two shirts, a pair of pajamas, a seersucker dress and a slip! And in Italy I paid 50 lire for everything every week, including a sheet and pillow case and four uniforms. Oh, well, I don't have anything else to spend my money on and I might just as well use it to be clean.

At eight o'clock I descend and find a tray set for me on the dining room table. Fatima, the Arab maid, is padding barefoot around the kitchen, Mme. Andre has already gone to work, but M. Andre is usually esconced in a big chair in the sun, reading the morning paper. Sometimes he has already eaten, sometimes he joins me for a cup of coffee, a bun sandwich which he makes out of the heel of the long brown loaf of French bread, cutting the thick heel in two and hollowing out a little place for a piece of cheese or a bit of meat left over from the night before, or sometimes he has a dish of soup, or sometimes he puts some cognac in his coffee. It is amazing what he will and does eat. I thought my cold baked potatoes took the prize, but M. Andre outdoes me.

He is never completely dressed at this hour, having on the top of his pajamas with his trousers and a pair of Arab slippers like those I sent you, Father, for Christmas. He is most talkative at this hour in the morning and as I said, I just sit there and smile and nod. My breakfast consists of a couple of cups of *café au lait*, sweetened with sugar that looks very much like our raw sugar, and a couple of pieces of dark bread, sometimes toasted, with honey or with sweet butter, or sometimes just plain. The enlisted man (I should say boy) who works with us bought me some oranges the other day, and I keep those in my room and eat one or two when I first get up in the morning, and some before I go to bed. Vitamin C is certainly not the one that is lacking from my diet. We get served orange juice at lunch here in the mess, and I frequently, if I can bribe with a smile the waiter, drink two or three glasses of it in lieu of coffee or wine or water. Makes me feel so healthy!

Yesterday after breakfast, M. Andre took me out to see the tremendous big artichokes he had brought in from the country: They were beautiful and I admired them so much that I was invited to come to dinner *en famille* today to eat some of them "cru." I wish I could, both come to dinner today and eat them raw. But the first I cannot accept because of our picnic, and the second wouldn't dare do. However, this morning I was given one of the biggest and best of the artichokes and I came to work carrying it like a bunch of flowers. What I will do with it now, I am not quite sure, but it is pretty to look at anyway.

Speaking of dining with them *en famille*, I have been very much accepted by the family now. The daughter has asked me to go out with her this afternoon on a party with some young French officers (an invitation which, malheuresment I cannot accept), Mme. Andre has asked me to have supper with the family once a week or so and talk English to the daughter (I don't believe I will be able to fit that in either, at least not for the time being), Mme. Andre has started to worry about the long hours I work, holding up her previous boarder as an example of overwork, telling me that he used to work late in the evenings and then got sick because he didn't get enough rest.

April 3, 1944

Yesterday, after I had admired the artichokes, we inspected the livestock. There is a big wire enclosure in the back yard with chickens and pigeons and rabbits in it. One of the rabbits was then expected to be confined very shortly (actually, it happened last night and just as I was going down the garden path this morning, Mme. Andre called to me in great excitement to come and see the ten little rabbits that had been born during the night. Ugly little things). M. Andre told me all about rabbits and pigeons and their peculiarities and I held one of the fairly recent rabbits in my arms, and the sun was warm, the sky blue, the pigeons every once in a while flew up over our heads with a whirr of wings, and everything seemed very right with the world. The French, particularly, *petit bourgeois* are a wonderful group. On Sundays they all get dressed up and go walking *en famille* in country and one meets them coming leisurely home at sunset, the baby asleep in Mother's arms, the children carrying big bunches of flowers and Papa with his coat flung over his shoulder, his shirt-sleeves rolled up, and a big cigar in his mouth. M. Andre is much more interested in his animals and his garden (he has many flowers, some fruit trees, and a big space for potatoes, string beans which are just coming up, carrots and other vegetables) than he is in the war. At least that is the impression that he gives. I have been given permission to pick any flowers I want for my *bureau* [office] and Mme. Andre keeps a vase of flowers fresh in my room. This morning I was give a packet of dates to take to work with me in case I got hungry during the day.

After the animals had been fed, I went back to my room and got ready to come to work. The first day, I made my bed quite automatically, but Mme. Andre was horrified and made me promise never to *déranger* myself again that way. So now I just hang up my pajamas and get my coat and take off. Peepo, the big police dog, took a few days to get used to me, but now he no longer barks when I come home at night, and yesterday when I opened the front door, there he was waiting on the doorstep for me. He politely got up when I came out, hesitated a moment and then obviously decided that I was an accepted member of the family and therefore should have suitable escort when I went out. So he walked just ahead of me all the way to work!

I get to the office just before nine and get things opened up for the day. Lunch is at 12, and supper at 7, and the hours in between are very full. I keep meeting people, either personally or hear about them, that I have known before, and it is a lot of fun.

Yesterday we had the mess put up our lunch for us and about seven of us went on a picnic. We didn't go far, about ten minutes away by car, but it was far enough for us to relax completely. The lunch wasn't too good, but we had a couple of bottles of wine, and sat on the grass, there was a little brook burbling down below us, there were hundreds of flowers of all sorts around us, and it was most pleasant and very good for us. We all worked much better in the afternoon because of the relaxation of the lunch hour. Does a dove make a noise like a cuckoo? We all of us heard the "cuckoo, cuckoo," but some people said it was a dove and some said a cuckoo.

April 15, 1944

Wonder of wonders, a quiet moment in the day's occupation! Of course, I really shouldn't even mention it, because that is usually the signal for riots to break out. But I'll keep my fingers crossed and get tomorrow's letter started today.

So many things are happening, that I hardly know where to begin to tell about them all. My work keeps on being time and energy consuming, and being as interesting as ever. I guess I am sufficiently of a romantic to be happy under these conditions. Anyway, I love it.

I'm so glad that Alex [de Bondini, whom I had met in Naples] wrote you so promptly. I had a simply wonderful afternoon with him—he is such a nice person. One amusing thing here is that I am working with a French-American officer, whom you may have met, who married the girl that Alex was at one time planning to marry. You have probably met her in New York, she is a good friend of Gregory's and used to go there often for dinner.

I am continually meeting people in this part of the world whom I know or else of whom I have heard a great deal. Makes things kind of fun....

I picked a big bunch of nasturtiums the other evening, just before supper, and it made me so homesick. I immediately wrote Doug to make sure that he had an old stone wall that I could cover with nasturtiums, *dopo la guerra*.

Mme. Andre finally get so worried about my not coming home in the afternoon, once a week as arranged, to take my bath, that she stopped me one evening as I was on my way up the stairs and told me that she had a heart, and that she couldn't bear to have me go dirty, (or words to that effect), that a pitcher of hot water every morning was not enough and that she was desolated that due to the war she had not been able to have a bidet installed in the little closet along with my washbasin, and that she herself would fix my bath for me the following morning at 7:30. She finally stopped talking long enough for me to tell her that she was too, too *gentile*, and that a bath would be *manifique*. So the following morning I had a wonderful, hot tub full of water in which to disport before breakfast. But the slight ring on the tub proved that I didn't need it as much as she insinuated!

This morning's breakfast was another one of those things. M. Andre was resplendent in blue pajamas, the works—no longer just the top with his trousers. The son had just received his promotion to the French equivalent of lance corporal, and they were joyful over that; the daughter's boy friend had apparently spent the night there, or else had just dropped in for an early breakfast—so to top the whole thing off, I was asked to dinner tonight, because they had just received a pig from the country. I accepted, not so much because I wanted to, but because I knew that it was inevitable that I must some time and I might just as well get it over with now. Then M. Andre thought perhaps I might prefer pigeon to pig; with due politeness I murmured that just anything would be all right. But to prove how nice pigeons were, Mme. Andre rushed out into the kitchen and brought back two plump ones, still warm, that M. Andre had killed just a short while before. I am sure that they were the ones that had preened themselves on the roof outside of my window a few mornings before, and now I had to touch them, assure Mme. Andre that I thought they would be delicious, and try not to think of eating them this evening. I managed to finish my *café au lait*, but then M. Andre desired to show to me the pig, which was in the scullery. So I was pushed out there, to admire a very large and dismembered and disemboweled carcass. Really, the French are just too frank and open about the less delicate sides of life. I am just waiting now for M. Andre to wake me up some morning to come out and see the rabbits mating or something!

Speaking of rabbits, most of the babies were killed by the mother. I told the Andres that as a child, I had had the same experience with my rabbits (remember the three I had, to teach me the facts of life, only all three had babies!). And that made me a kindred soul and they continued with great gusto to discuss the way pigs did the same thing. They don't mind *what* they talk about or when. It's amazing.

I finally, a shattered shell of my normal self, managed to escape down the garden path this morning, and had my morale considerably raised by the orange tree on one side of the gate, very fragrant in the early morning air, and the lilac tree on the other, just bursting into perfumed bloom. From the flat roof of the next house, a rooster lifted his voice like Chanticleer, to the newly risen sun, and paraded ostentatiously along the edge of the roof, back and forth silhouetted against the sky. I opened the gate, stepped out into the road, and stopped a minute to absorb the realization of what a beautiful day it was (in spite of pigs and pigeons) and a small, very clean and neat boy, carrying a basket full of long loaves of bread, smiled at me, said "Good morning" with a charming little accent, and extended his hand to shake hands with me. I was a little startled, as I had never seen the child before, but I shook hands with him and said "Bon jour", he asked me in French if my health was good, I assured him that it was and asked after his own. It too was good, we smiled gravely at each other and he passed on down the road, swinging slightly his basket of bread. It was one of the most curious things that have ever happened to me, sort of dream-like and unreal.

Oh, my—the mail boy just brought in a package for me. With that breathless Christmas or birthday feeling I opened it, fortunately in a corner because I had a slight recollection of some of the items you had included, Mother! Two slips, and a lovely blouse, and best of all some shoes! Whoopee! And Kleenex. And two more films. You are just wonderful, Mother. If now you can find someone to bring me a cotton dress or two your stock will be forever high. Today is so hot that we are just sitting around in this darned prefabricated hut and panting for air. The Sirocco has started extra early this year. I will be glad when we get our own villa and can move out of this hut. A tent would be better than this.

Mary Mock has been in town, my old boss from the 26th, and we had lunch together yesterday. But it was a little dis-appointing, as there was so little we could talk about.

A friend of mine will shortly be taking greetings to Richard [in England] and then a complete report to his par-ents. I'm trying to persuade him to take some oranges too. To Richard, I mean.

It's too hot to write any more now, and anyway I think I've about covered the subject. So I guess I will mail this a day early. By the way, this was not all written during that quiet (sic) interim this morning. Every hour on the hour all hell broke loose, or something. It seems a necessary con-comittant of this job that nobody does anything the quiet easy way, but always with as much rushing around and tele-phoning and noise as possible. So far I have managed to pur-sue my quiet way through the midst of the storm, gathering up as many of the loose ends as possible and straightening out what I can. It is kind of fun, and as long as I get a reasonable facsimile of enough sleep, I can manage.

My dinner with the Andres went much more smoothly than I'd anticipated. As I wrote home two days later, I admitted I'd really had a very good time.

My comprehension of French is really pretty good and after a glass of wine, I spoke reasonably fluently! We started out with an aperitif, then a delicious home-made soup, then a French version of the New England boiled dinner, which consisted of pieces of meat, fresh potatoes and carrots. Very good. Then the two pigeons, which I found I enjoyed very much in spite of my early morning introduction to them. And then a delicious salad right out of the garden around the house. I figured that it was as safe as any salad I could find over here, and I had eaten some under much less favorable circumstances and suffered no lasting ill effects. We had a fairly good vin rose with dinner, and for dessert sliced oranges with a wine sauce. Everybody was very gay, M. Andre told many funny stories, and it was very pleasant indeed.

I forgot to mention that before dinner, M. Andre had to show me the results of his day's work with the pig. Most of it had been salted away, sausages had been made and were hanging in the back yard, the kitchen was savoury with the *pate de foie* that Mme. Andre had been making, another pot had the beginning of head cheese in it, there was soup and stew and all sort of things (the origin of which I did not inquire into too carefully!). But I had maligned the boy who had breakfasted with us that morning, calling him the daughter's beau. It turned out that, young as he is (17), he is an excellent butcher. His father is a prisoner and he and his mother run between them a butcher shop. The mother takes care of business and the boy does all the butchering and cleaning and everything. So he had come in to help with day's work with the pig, or rather to direct it, I guess.

M. Andre's father, I discovered, lived in Carcasson, and was a skilled wood carver and did the carving on some panels or something in the Hotel de Ville there. They have photographs of them and they are really beautiful.

The family is really an interesting one, but you have never seen anything as funny as M. Andre in the mornings, still in his pajamas with a **beret** on and sometimes a sweater. It is wonderful. He absolutely adores his garden and the daughter says it almost takes a policeman to make him come in, even for meals.

In my last letter I forgot to tell you the high point of last week, which was meeting Marlene Dietrich! She was here on tour with the USO and we went to see her at the "Opera House" and afterwards went behind scenes to meet her. She is still beautiful, and still well. Remember how we used to play "Jonny" when my beaux came calling, just to watch their expressions? I thought I was too blasé or something to get a thrill out of meeting a "film star" but I was as excited as a high school girl.

Well, this is long enough for a supplementary letter. Thanks again for the packages.

I continued to emphasize on every possible occasion, however, that I considered my stay temporary. Its length would depend on how long it took to get my passport (which would be a diplomatic one assigning me to the embassy) and on the arrival of the promised additional secretarial help. Then I would move on to the assignment originally discussed when I resigned from the Red Cross.

April 22, 1944

First of all, Happy Birthday to you, Mother. I'm sorry that we haven't got better weather for you today, but perhaps you would like this sort of "open and shut" as much as I do. It is rather cozy to hear the rain on the roof, and my desk is right beside a little potbellied stove which casts a pleasant and relaxing warmth in my direction, and the wood smoke is heavenly. One of my jobs, since I am right beside the stove, is to bring in wood (when I can sneak past all the men who spring to their feet in horror when they see me doing any manual labor of any sort, except typing! Really, I have never been so sheltered and protected in my life. It is a bit amusing after the last fourteen months of sort of fending for myself. I get escorted everywhere, people apologize for slightly off-color stories, I mustn't lift anything heavy—it is very funny.)

From time to time the sun comes out, and the air is soft and fresh after the recent rain, and the leaves are shiny and wet and green and everything smells so nice. But the moisture in the air keeps the smoke from the little stoves hanging over the huts, and it smells like Chocorua [our family home in New Hampshire] on an early June morning, after rain.

My ego is inflated for good, beyond all pinpricks of future misfortunes. The way my services are being fought over! I am now being held for *two* secretaries, long expected. That is just silly, and as soon as *one* comes, I shall try to carry out my original plan. The various obstacles, like the far from enthusiastic greeting I got from our tall friend's colleague, only serve to make me more stubborn and insistent that I carry through my schedule. I may look like the docile type, but I can be very mule-like! [As if they didn't know.]

April 27, 1944

Some of my friends, colleagues of C [in Bari] have appeared here from time to time and the look of complete incredulity, surprise, and then (of course) pleasure which crosses their faces when they find me sitting at my desk here, is really most amusing. They are then a little likely to berate me for being a liar, but I think it is more a blow to their pride to find that beneath my "sweet and simple exterior" I was a little more complex than they had realized!

Goodness, I will be 27 next week, won't I? Must start looking for gray hairs!

Yesterday [Sunday] was a nice day, even though a long one, or perhaps *because* it was a long one. We all worked until 10:30 last night . . . but I liked it and didn't mind it at all that I had to break a date I had for cocktails and dinner with some people, among whom was the Major . . . the one who met you, Father, at the airport when you were visiting Alex [Kirk in Cairo].

April 30 was the "dark of the moon" and the reason for working so late might have been that we had gone out to the airfield to send off one of our agents to be dropped into France. I suspect that was what happened and it is one reason my letter the next day was so full of local color. It must have been extremely frustrating for me to have been unable to share with my parents those special and exciting events. I knew, however, that they did enjoy my descriptions of my surroundings, the more ordinary things I did, the people I saw, and I'm sure that the excerpts from my May 1 letter delighted them as much to receive as it obviously did me to write. Now, fifty years later, it brings back many vivid memories of sights and sounds and even smells.

Going to church had become a weekly routine, and, although I went into no detail about the service (perhaps because I knew it wouldn't interest them), I now find it very significant, in light of what I later realized was an ongoing spiritual journey.

Sundays I get up half an hour early and walk down the hill to the English church. It is a good half hour's walk, and is sometimes not only the only real exercise I get during the week but also the only time I get away from the immediate neighborhood of the office. I go down one little road, cut across an empty lot that is gay with flowers at this time of year, up a flight of steps, down another road and across a bridge, and then down a steep road that leads windingly down the hill. There are not many people up at this hour, just a few hurrying women on their way to early Mass, a few chattering American soldiers swinging their mess kits as they go down to relieve the night shift, and one or two Arab women clutching their robes around them as they patter along on their bare feet. A French boy scout, aged about twelve, tears pell-mell down the hill, running not because he is in a hurry but just for the sheer joy of speed and the wind in his face and the almost frightening feeling that one gets running downhill, one foot following the other always faster and faster until one has very little control over them at all. A sleepy dirty half-caste has opened the little kiosk in the square and has a dozen or so newspapers spread out for early morning buyers, the bakery is just opening its shutters, a lean and hungry dog noses the garbage out of the gutter.

Once on the steep hill road, one is shut away from the rest of the city by the high stone walls that rise on either side, with trees leaning over the top and occasional glimpses of gardens and villas through the open gates. The birds are just beginning to get into full tune and the trees are full of their twittering and chirping. One can hear the distant rattle of a tramcar, a jeep with some enlisted men I know toils up the road past me, but otherwise it seems a quiet and secret world of my own. One garden has been turned over to the Army and the tents are clustered incongruously in front of the villa. A quick but brief nostalgia for the freer life of tents over-comes me, and for a moment I am homesick for my tent, my cot, the outdoor life, the smell of the coffee in the morning and the rattle of mess kits and the call of the bugle. . . .

Down at the bottom of the hill, a short walk along a main street and there is the church. It is a very nice, plain one, the early service short, and the familiar ritual very soothing.

I get through just in time to catch the bus which brings me back in time to get breakfast here before going to work. I usually have a five-minute or so wait for the bus, and it is fun to see how much the city has waked up in the half-hour. I saw this last Sunday something I had not seen in a year and a half—someone posting a letter in a letter box! Funny, what a perfectly natural thing that is, and how strange it looked to me. For a minute, I couldn't figure out why it seemed so queer, and then I realized that it was because it had been so long since I had seen it.

The variety of uniforms is something marvelous to behold. There are many WACs here, and they look very efficient in either their neat skirts and blouses or their more prosaic "fatigues." I still get a kick out of seeing two girls driving up the street in a weapons carrier, both looking serious and purposeful, yet quite attractive. I even saw some driving trucks one day. Then there are the prim British WRENS, who belie their primness by the shortness of their skirts and the tremendous expanses of black-stockinged legs that appear. And the casual-looking British men, some of whom even this early are dressed in khaki shorts and bush jackets. And then my favorite yesterday was the very black boy, dressed in bright blue pants and jacket, with a bright red fez sort of cap perched jauntily on his kinky hair.

And of course there are an infinite number of variations in the Arab, even though his fundamental costume is the same. Degrees of cleanliness give the effect of completely different attire. The well-dressed, clean ones are very good-looking, their robes loose and flowing, their turbans bound neatly upon their heads and an air of dignity worn as an outer garment. But the beggar Arab is quite a different person, cringing and whining, dirty and ragged, with pride as much in tatters as clothes.

One of the most extraordinary sights is the North African equivalent of a Greyhound bus. A trolleycar is bad enough, simply bursting at the sides with the terrific load it carries, but the buses are out of this world, as the slang phrase goes. The baggage is heaped skyward on the roof, and the whole thing sways and tips in an alarming manner as it goes around corners. It puffs and chugs and creates an awfully smelly smoke, and one does not see how on earth it can go another twenty feet. Every possible square inch inside is jammed with people, Arabs and Europeans mixed together in a terrific *mélange*, with turbaned head close to felt hat, and white veil next to peroxide blond or violent red. The Arab men look strange enough, but the women seem completely out of place, their deep dark eyes peering out of the slit between veil and headdress.

I really have a tremendous liking for North Africa, and it will always be a very pleasant memory, the months I have spent here. This is the most beautiful part of the year, and the most pleasant. We went for a brief jeep ride in the country this afternoon, the poppies are just beginning to dot the fields with scarlet and the mountains are misty in the distance. Soon it will be too hot, but now is wonderful.

On May 9 I wrote a long letter home, the whole first page being about Doug, my feelings and my growing uncertainty about a future relationship with him. I wanted to be sure they weren't telling friends and relatives that I was "almost engaged to an Air Force officer whom I had met in Italy!" Some of my earlier letters had been so full of him and the time we'd had together and the things we'd done that I was afraid they might have jumped to what might prove erroneous conclusions! On a lighter note, I asked almost facetiously if Father thought there was any chance "Clover's husband," namely his longtime friend Allan Dulles, might need a secretary in Bern where he was OSS's chief of mission. "That might be quite a lot of fun."

Affairs of the heart and other miscellaneous items taken care of, I then went on to write more about my daily life.

We *déménaged* the other day to a villa, which makes a much more satisfactory office than the Army prefabricated hut we were in before. Much cooler and much more room, and much less confusion. Although to a stranger arriving in our midst the confusion would seem so great even here that he would find it hard to believe that there ever could have been more. As I wandered down the white and dusty road in the bright sunlight, carefully carrying a large vase of flowers to our new abode, I remembered other occasions when I had carried a bowl of goldfish or a lamp or something else equally conspicuous from one apartment to another in Brooklyn, the only difference—then I minded, now I don't.

Our villa gives me an opportunity to indulge in a little domesticity, on the side as it were. I take a merciless teasing about the flowers I am forever bringing in and arranging in vases. Frank [Schoonmaker, the head of the office and my boss] the other day threatened to throw them all out as I had used all the pitchers and half the water glasses, and he wanted a glass or two for drinks! And when I told him that Fitzgerald [another member of the staff] was buying me some vases in town, he wanted to know why I didn't get a tub while I was at it. But in spite of everything, I continue. And it does make the house look better. This morning I have one big vase full of red poppies and various seed grasses, another with field flowers, a lovely bouquet of roses on the hall table (contributed by M. André and by the family across the road from us). And Theo [an office colleague] has a glass of odds and ends on her desk, and I have some pansies, some yellow iris, and some grasses on my desk. (Make you sneeze to think of it, Father?)

And before we got our mess set up and were cooking on a single electric hot plate, I cooked lunch for the boys a couple of days, making scrambled eggs and toasted tomato and bacon sandwiches and Nescafé. I started to shell peas on the front porch one afternoon, just for the fun of it, but Frank came along and looked very pained and asked me if I *insisted* on doing that, so I stopped and let the kitchen boys do it. Apparently it was behavior not acceptable for a secretary, even if at the moment she had nothing to do, and wanted to shell peas. So I guess I'll have to wait until I get back to

Chocorua, and then I shall shell all the peas that I want. May I?

Fascinating country this—one hears a strange noise and looks up to see a herd of cows gently ambling down the road past one's window, and a few minutes later a whole herd of goats skitters by followed by a ragged urchin of an Arab child, sex indeterminate because of dirt and tatters and tender age.

The most pleasant events of the weeks now are the long walks I take with a most congenial captain [an office colleague]. Two or three times a week we meet after supper and spend a couple of hours roaming the hills and paths of the neighborhood, until darkness sends us home again. These walks are the source of most of my flowers, and I come home laden down with my gatherings. Last evening was cool and a little misty, a pleasant change from the previous day's *sirocco*. We started off down a macadam road, but soon cut off on a dirt road, then across a field and then up a hill via a little goat path. He knows how to walk and doesn't stop for silly things like helping me up over a stone wall. We walked through vineyards that are as yet just green sprouting stumps, past orchards heavy with the small green fruit and scarlet with poppies underneath, over gentle hills and down into shallow valleys, glancing through the dooryards of Arab hovels and French farmhouses—alike only in the barking dog that marked our passing. My hands got fuller and fuller of flowers, each field that we passed had something new that I wanted to add to my collection—poppies and blades of green wheat, the pink mallow, yellow iris, pale pink wild roses, magenta flags. We got farther and farther away, each winding road seemed to beckon us, each cloud wrapped hill looked inviting. It got darker as dusk crept around us and we finally decided that we had better find our way home. But the roads were by now unfamiliar and they seemed to lead us farther away from the direction in which we thought we ought to go. A friendly farmer told us that the path through his farmyard led to the main road, and as we went by we admired his low rambling house and the rose gardens on the terrace below, and the subsequent terraces with vegetables and then orange trees. The path zigzagged back and forth down into the valley and then wound back up the other side through his vineyards. But still we did not recognize our surroundings. Another farmyard, another country lane and a passing Arab, noting our hesitation, offered to show us the shortcut back to the section from which we had come. Much to our delight, the shortcut took us through an Arab cemetery, the white marble of the strange tombs very ghostly in the twilight. The lights were on now in the houses of the countryside and they sparkled and twinkled in the Scotch mist. Twice more we asked directions, still we did not know just where we were. Then, to my giggling astonishment, we came out just below where I live. All the time we had been almost within a stone's throw of familiar territory! But it was fun, good exercise, pleasant company, and I had my armful of flowers.

My next letter, typed on one of those difficult-to-decipher V-mail forms, described some of my extra-secretarial duties. On May 18 I wrote that I gave

advice to the lovelorn, treated several people for dysentery, was general buffer and pacifier and soother of ruffled tempers and deflated egos and supervised the mess (meaning of course the cooking and eating facilities, not "disorder" though I'm sure that was also part of the problem). I have a complete medical kit now (where on earth did I get that?) and can dose and bandage to my heart's content.

I guess I hadn't completely gotten over my earlier dreams of becoming a doctor. And I ended by writing that

things are marching slowly but if Mrs. Shipley [head of the State Department Passport Division in Washington] crashes through soon, as she should, I hope things will be settled within ten days or two weeks. I expect to spend the next week training the two girls who were due yesterday. Much as I am enjoying this, I have had almost enough and am awaiting my release with ill-concealed impatience.

However, two days later I learned that once again the plans were delayed, this time because neither of the two girls, though classified as secretaries, could take shorthand and only one could type! And it was obvious, therefore, that I would have to stay on a bit longer. SNAFU again—but realizing that didn't make it any easier to accept.

I had simmered down a bit by the time I wrote on May 22:

Giving advice seems to be the biggest of my jobs here (even though it isn't in my job description!). I spend my days juggling the varied personalities with whom I have to work, acting as buffer between the conflicting ones. It is impossible to get a moment to myself, except in the bathroom, for no matter where I am, the others just seem to gravitate there too. I tried tonight, as I have before, to leave the dinner table a little early, while the others were having their coffee, so that I might be alone (like la Dietrich) for a few minutes (come to think of it, it is Garbo, isn't it). But I had been in my office not even five minutes when one of the boys drifted in with his unfinished glass of beer. A few minutes later another one wandered by the open door and ended up sitting on the couch, and finally the third one joined us, leaving those two new secretaries of ours sitting by themselves in the dining room. And yesterday I went into Frank's room to lie down for a half hour after lunch and take a nap, as I had been a bit shortchanged on sleep the night before, but I forgot to lock the door and shortly I had half the staff in there with me, sitting on the edge of the bed. Everybody brings me their problems, either personal or business, and I feel like a strange combination of mother, sister and sweetheart to half a dozen men. And I thought that the Red Cross was emotionally exhausting! It was a picnic in comparison. I only hope that I can keep the varied love lives straight and not ask the wrong one about the wrong girl or situation. I even got a sort of proposal the other night. The guy was tight, but I am afraid he meant it, and he wanted me to keep him next on the list if ever I changed my mind about Doug. It makes, as you might guess, for a rather delicate situation from the job point of view. But so far my juggling has been successful and I try not to play favorites.

Now that we have our own villa, we maintain our own mess, and we have obtained [General Henri] Giraud's former chef, complete with tall pleated white hat, to cook for us. Poor thing, the kitchen is little more than closet size and the stove smokes on windy days and someone is always forgetting to get him wood and the rations are usually late— how or why he stands it I don't know, except maybe these crazy Americans amuse him. We are able to supplement the Army rations with many other things in the way of fish and vegetables and fruit, and with Frank choosing the wine, it is far superior to that served in the regular mess. Frank's ambition is to have the best mess in town, and maybe he will. [After the war Frank Schoonmaker headed a prominent wine importing company.] It is all right with me! One thing, this war has not ruined my appetite, but it does amuse me to hear people fussing about the food, when it is so much better, even without the chef, than what I had eaten for the last fourteen months. They should try living on Spam and C rations for a while!

Just got interrupted to put some Argyrol into someone's eyes. And a few minutes ago the problem was where to get some fish for lunch. Never a dull moment, as I have said. And the little girl from the laundress has quite a crush on me and will not do business with anyone else! So no matter whose laundry it is, I have to go out and get it and settle the bill with her. What a life and what a war.

Much love,
Elizabeth

Two days later:

I have a few free minutes, so I will get a start on tomorrow's letter, and see if this week I cannot get it out on time.

I suppose I should be annoyed at a job that keeps interfering with my social engagements. I make very few dates, for several good reasons, and schedule a certain number of evenings in the office anyway, but last night and tonight both I have had to call up and break dinner dates. Tonight was for my date with Edouard [my very first beau at age 16 in New Hampshire]. He had suddenly appeared out of my past at a dinner party in Algiers and I had, partly out of curiosity, agreed to go out with him one evening, so I told him I would meet him later. It is funny, but it gives me a curious satisfaction to be able to say that I am unexpectedly tied up until 9:30 so that I won't be able to keep the dinner date. I suppose partly it makes me feel important, yet conversely I get pleasure out of the fact that there is something bigger than my own personal plans; perhaps that is what the psychiatrists call identification.

My own social life has amused me a little . . . I don't go out very much and it took me some time to make friends here out of the office. But now that I have established my own sort of set, it turns out that I know some of the "best" people, the most interesting and the most useful. "Ask Lee" has become the stock phrase, if anyone wants anything or wants to meet someone. It is quite fun. I proved my reputation was not just an idle one when the other night one of our new girls wanted to see her fiancé, who was here for just a short time. I said I was sure I could fix her up. We took her to the villa where some of my friends live and one of them went to call an influential and high-ranking personage who said why that must be Doctor So-and-So, of course she must see him. And she did. (Just between you and me, I was as impressed with the results of my social relationships as everyone else was.) I got a bit of vicarious pleasure out of bringing the two together, even for that short time, and hoped that someday someone would do as much for me!

The non-rationed black sandals did wonders for my morale. I had forgotten what fun it is to wear shoes with silly bows on them, and what fun it is to wear clothes that are not just practical and. . . .

May 29, 1944

I knew that would happen—but anyway I got one page written. . . . What started all that was that I love my new clothes and am ever and ever so grateful to you both for having such good taste, for getting them so promptly and for sending them to me.

Yesterday was a lovely peaceful day. In the morning I spent a whole hour sitting on the front porch in the sun, rereading *The Nutmeg Tree*, and interrupted only by our little Arab maid who brought a gigot of lamb for me to approve of (I tried to look very professional as I held it up and inspected it), by the chef who wanted to know if I thought the cherries were all right for dessert, and by one of our enlisted men who had cut his finger and wanted it bandaged! Just a nice quiet hour! Then in the afternoon we went for a short drive, and last night I went to the opening dinner of the Officers' Rest Camp on the seashore. A beautiful place, but too many people. The longer I stay overseas, the more certain I am that there are too many people in this world, and my idea of what I want to do first when I get home is to be ALONE. Most of my friends want to see all their other friends or get tight or spend a whole week going to all the night clubs and what have you in New York. But me, (and they all think I'm crazy) I want to go to Chocorua and not see anyone for ten days. Just sleep and be by myself and take hot baths and lie in the sun and eat millions of fresh vegetables and drink quarts of milk. Family, of course, doesn't count as people, and if Doug wanted that sort of thing, he could come along too. But I am not sure that he would. He might, though.

I got out my blue bead [a Turkish good-luck charm given

to me by a friend in Istanbul] the other day and rubbed it, like Aladdin's lamp, in the hope that that would do some good. I am fighting pretty much a lone battle here on that matter [of pursuing reassignment]. Absolutely everyone is opposed to it, as far as I can see, and it is a bit discouraging. They cannot see why I am so anxious to follow through the original plan and try to persuade me with all sorts of foolish reasons, like the so-called gayer life here, the more congenial people here, the more interesting events. If it were not for your so positive statements to the contrary, Father, they might have succeeded, but my confidence in your judgment, (at least as far as this is concerned!), is unshaken.

Another five-page letter written on June 5, mostly about odds and ends, finished with a description of a more interesting expedition:

A couple of Sundays ago we took a long ride, on official business, into the country and I saw my first camels for many months. They are, I think, one of my favorite animals, and it was fun to see them again. Some were completely hidden under tremendous loads of green branches, one was tethered in solitary splendor in the midst of a big field, and others were just ambling along the road. They are put together in such a wonderful way, their big squashy feet sort of like a cocker spaniel pup's and their incredibly long eyelashes which give them such a supercilious look, and their long noses which should have lorgnettes perched on them.

During the afternoon I had to wait in the car, which was parked in the yard of a French villa, for about twenty minutes. Farmyard would be a better description of it, for it was surrounded with barns and chicken yards and such. One's first impression was one of sun, dust and flies, children, chickens and dogs, all in a welter of confusion. The children, chickens and dogs vanished as we drove up, but curiosity brought them out again very shortly, as soon as I had been sitting there quietly for a few minutes. The little Arab children were an unbelievable collection of rags and tatters and dirt, and two small boys decided to attract attention to themselves by fighting in the dust. It was put on at first, but their imagined grievances reminded them of real ones and the rough-house turned into a strangely quiet, curiously adult circling around each other with an occasional cuff or kick and with Arab imprecations muttered at each other under their breath. A dozen or so other children appeared from nowhere and watched for a while and then went about their own games and pastimes, until Papa came along, a very jaunty young Arab, and separated the youngsters—one reverted to his age and retired into a corner weeping and the other looked at me smugly and with a sort of spoiled-son expression on his face. Most of the group were boys, the girls even at a tender age are kept in the compound and expected to help with the women's work. Every once in a while one would come down the path carrying a battered pail on her head, which she would fill at the pump and lug up the hill again. The Arab women definitely lead the harder life and the men loaf around, smoke and drink coffee all day long. The aristocrats of the race may be fine people, but the hangers-on in town or the suburbs are far from admirable.

One other strange custom that I have forgotten to tell you about—here where goat's milk is needed for more than the kids [baby goats]. The kids are either bitted with a small wooden bit or a loose string muzzle, or the mother's bag is enclosed in cloth so that the kids cannot nurse. It gives a strange appearance to them, like a skirt hanging down underneath.

Here comes the mail courier, and I want to get this out.
Much love to you all,
Elizabeth
(Hope you don't have to pay extra postage!)

It seems odd, fifty years later, to realize that D-Day made so little impression on me that I made no reference to it in this letter. It may have been that we were so concentrated on and involved in activities in southern France that what was happening in England and northern France didn't seem noteworthy.

June 11, 1944

This will be a pretty cheerful letter because so many nice things have happened this last week.

First, I have finally got a competent secretary to help me and to train to take my place! We stole her from another job which did not half keep her busy, and now she is easing my burden and amusing us all. She is very attractive and gay and efficient, even takes some dictation in French, so she is a great addition. So now Mrs. Shipley [the passport lady] is the only person who is holding me back, and I persuade someone to send a cable on that matter practically every other day. I expect everything will take three or four weeks yet, but I have hopes of carrying through our original plans the first part of next month. You don't know how I am look-ing forward to it, sort of a safe port after a stormy and very tempestuous voyage. When I was back home I used to look for jobs with lots of variety and aspects—now to my weary mind a straight secretarial job with nothing but shorthand, typing and filing seems ideal! All this extracurricular stuff is exhausting me. I left the Red Cross because I was tired of the constant drain on my emotions; here it is far worse. Everybody has the temperament of an opera singer and must constantly be soothed and reassured and pampered. And that is my job. I suppose I might just as well get used to the idea that people always will come to me with their problems and troubles and questions—I seem to be by nature a sort of Dorothy Dix (a syndicated good-advice columnist). Any-thing that needs to be done, and anything that anyone needs, it is always "Ask Lee." Perhaps I should be flattered, but frankly, I am just tired.

Reading this now, I wonder whether it was my 'satiable curiosity' like that of Kipling's "Elephant Child" that led to my willingness to listen to other people's problems and try to help them out. Or was it perhaps an early indication of my later vocation to the ordained ministry? Naturally I prefer the second interpretation.

The new secretary's advent will also result in a short vacation for me this coming week and a day off a week from now on. I have just called and made my reservations at the hotel on the beach, that I háve mentioned before, for Tuesday, Wednesday and Thursday nights. I shall take a couple of books and some olive oil and go into seclusion for three whole days. Lovely idea. Perhaps I shall be social at night, especially as there is a dance there Wednesday night, but the rest of the time I shall be very anti-social, if I can. And fortunately, my bathing suit arrived yesterday. I think I shall give you a medal, Mother, as being the most successful shopper for an absent daughter that anyone ever knew. I don't see how you do it; I don't believe I could do as well myself for myself. The bathing suit is perfect, color, size and fit. Absolutely wonderful, in fact. The shorts are a little big, but they can easily be fixed. And the material is so very pretty. I shall save it and try a different school of dressmaking for it. And I loved all the "findings" and the dye and the knife. The latter was particularly welcome because a French colonel friend of the Andrés was very anxious to get a knife and the P.X. hasn't got them any more. So I gave him the one I have been using, which is a fairly heavy one, and I shall keep the Girl Scout one for myself. I suppose when I get home I shall have to break myself of the habit of carrying around things like flashlights and knives and such. Over here I have gotten used to being prepared for anything at all times.

I also got today a charming note from our tall friend [my hoped-for next boss] and from his secretary. Very heart-warming, both of them, and very cordial. I shall be glad when all this uncertainty is over and I can settle down more or less. I am even a little journey-proud at the moment. People are beginning to accept it here and the opposition is melting and help is even being offered. So I am quite happy about the whole thing, at last.

The letters from "Our tall friend" and his secretary in the OSS Madrid office had reached me by diplomatic pouch. Before I could send them on to my parents via ordinary mail I had to censor them to delete the names of people and places. Thus

June 5, 1944

Dear Elizabeth,

Thank you so much for your letter of May 18, which is the first word which I have received on the rather confused subject of your final destination. It is useless at the moment to go into the details [illegible] which have been exchanged between . . . [censored] on a triangular circuit and direct, discussing your assignment. All I need say is that we need you here and are looking forward to having you join us just as soon as [censored] and our other friends are able to release you. I understand that [censored] must still rely heavily upon you for its stenographic work.

Not being able to speak very authoritatively in *loco parentis*, I have turned over that part of your letter which concerns clothes and such to [censored] who will add a note making the suggestions which appear to be most practical.

I thoroughly agree that the time you have spent in North Africa cannot be considered as wasted, and you will undoubtedly be most valuable to us in that you will have a better knowledge of actual conditions in [censored] than any of our staff here.

I understand that your Father is now in New Hampshire for two or three weeks of well-earned rest and the usual chores connected with the opening of the Chocorua house. I thoroughly miss his genial letters while he is away from work, but look forward to a continuation of our correspondence, I hope at a time when I can tell him that we have been fortunate enough to have you join us.

Yours sincerely,

[censored]

June 7, 1944

Dear Elizabeth

[Censored] has asked me to drop you a note about the questions in your letter, but before I start that, I want to tell you how much we're looking forward to your coming here. . . .

The only things I would suggest bringing with you are your Red Cross uniform, which seems to me with the insignia removed would look like any other suit, unless the mark where the insignia was is so plain that you wouldn't want to wear it as a suit, and the topcoat, which undoubtedly is not much different from most sport topcoats. It seems to me that you would not go wrong in packing your stuff in something like a duffel bag, as that is what many people do who come over here.

You won't have any use here for such items as mosquito nets, messkit, canteen and blankets, so it hardly seems worth the trouble of bringing them along.

One thing which no one may have told you is that practically anything you need can be bought in [censored], although prices are high, so I'm sure that you will have no trouble at all getting along until you can get your things from home . . .

On June 11, I went on a vacation at a nearby beach hotel. Then:

18 June 1944

Well, here I am back from my "vacation" a little browner and a little more rested, but more loath than ever to cope with the personality problems here.

Wednesday morning I ate breakfast at the last possible moment, 9 o'clock, a very uninspired typically Army meal, and then adjourned to the terrace in my smart new green playsuit, with my recently arrived *Mademoiselle* and *Cosmopolitan* under my arm. There I basked in the sun and window-shopped in the ads until lunch time, a meal which was much better than breakfast. After lunch I attired myself in my stylish new aqua and white bathing suit, thoroughly covered myself in olive oil (so that I smelled quite like a salad) and laden with towels, shirt, books, bandanna and such, descended to the beach.

By four o'clock the beach looked just like a nice private beach at home, with bevies of beautiful girls dressed in not much at all, dozens of darkly tanned young men, and even a couple of lifeguards (who spoiled the illusion if you spoke to them, as they answered in Italian) and a tall white stand for them to sit on. It seemed incredible that this was war, even though the morning had reminded us all of that fact. I forgot to mention that all morning long airplanes had been target-practicing on a large rock out to sea, and the air had been noisy with the chatter of machine guns over the rock and the louder crump of bombs which they dropped all around it. First there would be the sound of the plane, flying very low, then the white curl of water and smoke as the bomb hit—the white plume drifting up in slow motion, curling over itself until sometimes it left a perfect circle in the middle, a clear space through which one could see the blue water beyond. And then, a bit later, the noise caught up with the rest of the picture. Sometimes two planes would come out together and just play around in the sky, swooping and darting, until one wondered whether they were copying the swallows that darted out from the eaves of the house, or whether the swallows were imitating them. Then finally, just to completely destroy the illusion of peace and quiet, the guns on the shore did some target practice on a target drawn behind a plane. That made a terrific noise, but it was fun to watch how close they came to the target and to see the bright flash in the air and the little puff of white smoke afterwards. But those of us on the terrace decided that definitely it was no place to send someone with shell shock!

Mail has been coming through pretty quickly, although I think there have been gaps. Father's letter of June 11th came the 17th! The pictures I love—particularly Father and the flowers. I sent that one and the one of Mother watering the flowers to Doug! I thought he should have some idea of what he might be getting into! He is not to keep the pictures, though, just look and return, as I wouldn't be without them for anything. . . .

On June 20 I wrote, "Mrs. Shipley finally crashed through," meaning my passport and travel orders were being issued. A formal letter to me confirming this from G. Howland Shaw, Assistant Secretary of State, caught up with me later. With my departure finally official and documented, I had to tell my French family that I would be leaving soon. As I wrote home on June 26:

The atmosphere *chez André* is rather sad these days. I had dinner with them Saturday night and halfway through the meal I broke the news to them that I was not a permanent boarder. There was stunned silence for a minute, but they are well brought up and did not pester me with questions. M. André wanted to know who was going to bring me roses in the morning. Mme. André wanted to know if I thought I might be near Doug. And then they brought out the last bottle of Benedictine which they had been saving for the 14th of July and we solemnly toasted each other. The party got a little merrier after that. M. André promised to come to the States after the war. Mme. André said she hoped he would change his costume before he went (he had on his favorite gardening trousers, faded blue with dark blue patches on each knee and a big one in the back. I love them myself.) Then the other guest, a charming little-more-than-middle-aged man who has some important government position, and who looks a little bit as Fred Astaire might look in another fifteen or twenty years, did a tap dance and song act for us in the doorway of the living room. And we all sang songs. They brought out another bottle of a plum liqueur, colorless and very dry (and not too good to my taste). We drank some more and sang some more and it was really very pleasant. I shall miss "my" family very much. My three months with them have been very happy and they have filled an emotional need. They have, of course, completely spoiled me.

Walking to work the other morning a worried little Arab boy stopped me to ask if I had seen his black goat. I wanted to say yes, but I really hadn't seen it so I couldn't reassure him and he went on up the road, looking very ragged and anxious.

Patsy's father [General Donovan, head of OSS] was here for a few days and put us all into a frenzy of cleaning and straightening up. I don't remember him at all. I had thought perhaps when I saw him again he would look familiar. He seems like a pleasant enough person, but I didn't have a chance to talk to him at all, so beyond that I could not venture an opinion.

I am getting more and more journey-proud, and have spent part of the morning typing a list of useful words and phrases to help me with any linguistic problems. My emotions seem to be a mixture of excitement, a little being scared, and a tremendous anticipation. Seems almost impossible that at last it is coming to pass. It has certainly taken a long time.

Sleepily, but much love,

As I had written earlier, Doug had finally received his orders to go back to the States on compassionate leave because of his father's serious illness. Thus for all practical purposes ended the part of my life called "Doug." It was wonderful while it lasted but as I had phrased it , "love grows rapidly in the hothouse of strange times, places and circumstances...." I reassured my parents that if it turned out to be just a wartime romance I would not go into a convent or a Victorian decline. I have many happy memories and still remember him with real affection.

One last sort of winding-up letter was written a day later:

One of the hardest things I ever did was this last week of completely delegating the responsibility to the new secretary. I sat out in the other room and at times had to sit on my hands and bite my tongue to keep from interfering and reminding her of things. But it seemed to me the only way for her to learn what it was all about was to turn it all over to her and get her to call for help when and if she needed it. And, equally, I had to teach Frank to holler for her instead of for me. But it took a good deal of self-discipline to sit idle and never offer anything, just wait until I was asked.

I am afraid that time is too short and the evening too late for me to tell you all about the Arab dinner the Andrés took me to last Sunday.

The dinner that I can tell you about is the one the Andrés gave me last night. Cream of spinach soup, fresh shrimp salad, the shrimps for which M. André drove out to get himself, leg of lamb (the lamb had been killed especially in my honor) grilled tomatoes and squash, straw potatoes, green salad, baked peaches, cake with chocolate filling, chocolate cream, *infusion de vervaine avec du rhum*, and crème de menthe! It was a gay but sad party. They gave me a pin painted with roses to remind me of the roses M. André gives me every morning, and I felt as if I were saying goodbye to my family all over again. Do write them if you have the time, Mother. They have been so darling to me. Mme. André gave me two bunches of lavender to put with my clothes. She does all my laundry now, she dyed two of my gray dresses (I have on the lavender one now and it is very pretty). She had someone practically remake some of my underwear—I cannot begin to tell you all the nice things they have done.

I am too tired to write more tonight. Perhaps more in a different setting tomorrow night.

So ended another chapter and I left for Madrid at last, on Sunday, July 9, 1944. I still have that pin painted with roses, wear it occasionally, and treasure the inscription on the back: "To Miss Lee Phenix with our best wishes, The Andrés."

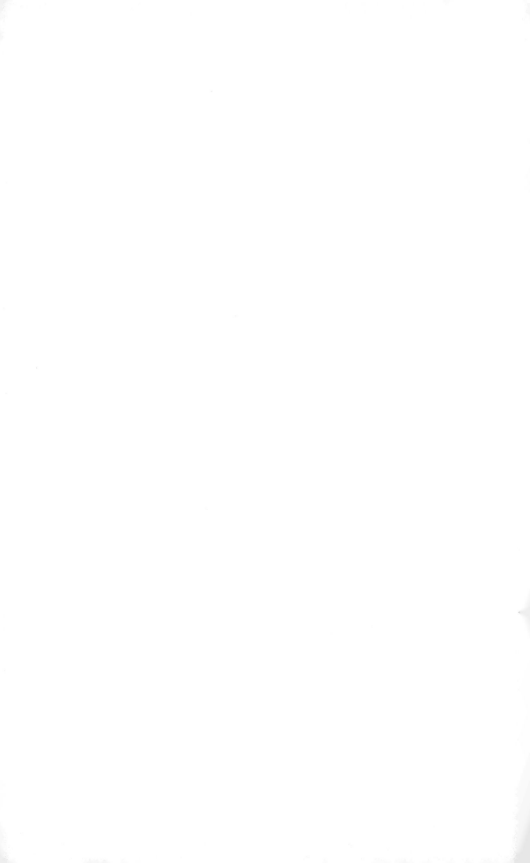

CHAPTER FIVE

Have Passport, Will Travel

—❖—

July 9–September 25, 1944

On July 20 a group of high ranking German military officers, tried to assassinate Adolf Hitler. The attempt failed and most in the plot—including Field Marshal Erwin Rommel—were executed, thus ending the only credible opposition in Germany to the Führer.

Soviet troops crossed into Poland on July 27. Five days later Warsaw rose against the Germans in a heroic two-month effort, but Stalin cynically halted the Red Army's advance, thus sacrificing the patriotic Poles.

The U.S. Seventh Army landed in southern France August 15 and began moving up the Rhone Valley. French troops took Marseilles August 23. Paris was liberated August 25 after four years of Nazi occupation, and General Charles de Gaulle entered the city in triumph. Antwerp fell to the Allies September 4, Brussels on September 5.

Rocket-powered buzz bombs and V-2s, Germany's new weapons of terror, took a rising toll in Britain, despite Allied bombing of launch sites and factories.

A World Monetary and Financial Conference in July at Bretton Woods, New Hampshire, established the International Bank for Reconstruction and Development (World Bank) and the International Monetary Fund (IMF).

Travel I did, although without a passport for almost three months. In the meantime, someone somewhere provided me with the necessary travel orders which enabled me to leave Algiers by plane on July

137

9. In Madrid I was given a document with a wonderful red seal identifying me as *a Functionaria del Gobierno de los Estados Unidos de America asignada a esta Embajado* and signed by Findley Burns, Secretary of Embassy. The worn condition of this document and its envelope clearly indicates that I carried it with me everywhere.

My first letter home, dated July 17, was to my mother as my father was still traveling. Incredibly, and to my delight, his itinerary included Spain and he had been able to spend some time in Madrid shortly after I arrived; our reunion was as much fun as the earlier one in Algiers.

Dear Mother:

I left a week ago yesterday morning with very few regrets I must admit. A Major friend escorted me to the airport, having picked me up at my house at some early hour (the Andrés hadn't known that I was going so early and trooped downstairs in various stages of undress to say goodbye to me—and M. André rushed around the garden to pick me my last bouquet of roses, Mme. André trying to hide her tears. It was really very touching and I almost cried too).

I had, as usual, much too much baggage but the Major promised to get it all on for me, even if he had to say it was unclaimed luggage being returned to Gib [Gibraltar]. That was not necessary, as the young British lad who weighed it in was in a sympathetic mood and added to my allowance and the rest to my personal weight. So the weight manifest had me down as weighing 195 lbs! Not only did this get my stuff on board but it served as an introduction to the South African crew who kept peering out of their compartment forward, in eager curiosity to see the girl who weighed so much. We started to take off when they decided one of the engines wasn't quite right, so everybody got off for another cup of tea while the mechanics tried to fix it. The navigator, South African like the rest of them, was very un-British in his forwardness in asking me to join him, so the captain, the co-pilot, the flight sgt. and the navigator and I all had tea together and they confessed their curiosity about my avoirdupois, and I confessed my conspiracy with the chap who weighed me in. It was the beginning of a very pleasant friendship, for as soon as the plane (a different one, they couldn't fix the first one) took off I was invited forward; followed by the envious glances of my fellow passengers, I forsook the uncomfortable bucket seats, picked my way over the freight and through the door that said "No Admittance to Passengers" into the crew compartment. They put me in the co-pilot's seat and handed me the weather reports as they came in, and explained everything to me, and in general made the time pass very quickly. When we landed for lunch, they insisted that I would not get enough to eat in the lunchroom where the others ate, so I was taken into the kitchen and well fed. On the next leg of the flight I again sat forward, this time in the pilot's seat, and they tried to persuade me not to get off at Gib but to continue with them. At one time it was thought that the wind would be too great to allow us to land, and they were overjoyed. But I was much relieved when we made a perfect three-point landing.

The courier met the plane (we were several hours late so the military attaché from the consulate had not been able to wait), my myriad pieces of luggage were collected, the navigator took me for a last cup of tea and asked me to write him, and the first lap of my journey was over. We went first to the consulate, where I paid my respects to the military attaché (whose brother was in Father's class at Harvard) and then up to the Rock Hotel. My name had come through as Captain Phenix, for some reason, so we discovered that I was supposed to share a room with a wing commander. However, they wouldn't even let me see what sort of a guy he was, but right away insisted on other accommodations. All that was available was the sitting room belonging to the manager, a sort of Mr. Milquetoast individual who gathered his tea things to his bosom when I came in and scuttled out in a rabbity fashion. I am sure that his reputation is ruined (or made, depending on how you look at it) because I could never remember what the room number was and when asked what room I was in, would airily reply that I was staying with the manager.

I luxuriated in a warm bath, first having had tea sent up, then Fred (the courier) came after me and we went down to the military attaché's room for a drink and then had dinner together. The ambassador's secretary, named Michael, joined us and after dinner the colonel took us in his car on a trip around the rock, to the Yacht Club for a dance or two, and then back to the big and shadowy terrace of the hotel for a beer before we went to bed. The dream really started then, I think, and as yet I have not waked up, and there seems little chance that I will as long as I am here.

The next morning we explored the town and did a little shopping—I bought a very nice pair of low-heeled black suede shoes, British, for a very reasonable sum. Good for next winter! Fred was supposed to drive me up but the amount of my baggage worried him and he had a lot of official stuff, so I was turned over to Michael. It was quite a blow to my *amour propre* that he was not more enthusiastic about the prospects of my company, but I later found out why. He is really part of the family here at the embassy and he had overheard part of a lecture that Mrs. Hayes [the ambassador's wife] gave her daughter once on the appearances of a young man and a girl traveling together, and he was very much concerned over her reaction when she discovered that we had been together on such a trip with only the dubious chaperonage of the chauffeur! She did hear about it, of course, and it was she who told me with much amusement why it was that Michael had been so reluctant, and we laughed together about it.

We left Gib shortly after noon, without lunch, and stopped about four o'clock (Spanish style) to eat at a wonderful sort of inn at a place called Torremolinos, right on the edge of the sea. After the sort of food that one gets in restaurants in North Africa and after the not-so-good food at Gib, the meal was pure ambrosia and the place so charming that Michael and I decided it was the perfect place for a vacation. That makes three ideal places I now know—Carmel in California, Amalfi in Italy, and Torremolinos in Spain (how I do get around!). We tore ourselves away about 5:30 and continued our drive, up across the coastal mountains and away from the sea. It is impossible to give you all the details of the trip—the car is the ambassador's own, very luxurious and with an American flag in front. Soldiers along the road saluted, laborers touched their caps—I felt as if I should blow kisses to the children or toss pennies to the villagers. A trifle different from the jeeps that I am accustomed to as a mode of travel. Getting through customs, something that had worried me a bit with my complete ignorance of the language, was of course no problem at all. Traveling *diplomatico,* they never opened a bag. And Michael speaks very good Spanish, so I had no worries whatsoever. He gradually relaxed and, I guess, decided not to worry about the appearances and my conversation was sufficiently foolish so that he was half convinced that I wasn't too bright anyway. It took him a good half day to figure me out—I would startle him with questions like "In Madrid does one mix socially with the Germans?" [Spain was officially neutral in World War II.] But we got along together very well, he is the kind of person one can be quiet with as well as talk, and I think he got quite a kick out of my obvious delight and enjoyment of the whole trip.

Next chapter—my night at Grenada, the gypsies and what they foretold.

21 July 1944

Dear Mother:

To get back to my saga. Michael and I got to Grenada about 9:30 that night, just as the sun was setting. The hotel is halfway up a hill, so that it overlooks part of the city and the wide plain beyond. Michael's confusion was further augmented by the desk clerk asking if we wanted a double or twin beds! With a little difficulty we got separate rooms and I went up to bathe and change, and to stand on the balcony for a few minutes and admire the view. Then I joined Michael on the terrace where he was sitting with a couple of people from the embassy, also on their way back to Madrid. One of them, Dick, went to college with Dave Flaccus [a friend in New Hampshire] and to Georgetown with Paul DuVivier [whom I met first in Paris the summer of my freshman year]. So we felt like old friends right away. Michael had to leave shortly to pay his respects to the British consul, and the others had some sort of engagement, so they left after making sure that I was happily surrounded by drinks, salad, cold meat and rolls. It was very nice and peaceful there on the terrace with the stars coming out, the faint noises of the city below me, and a gentle breeze coming off the mountains at the left. Just as I was really relaxing, Michael dashed back to say that he had met the other two in town and that they had arranged for a gypsy dance and would we come? Poor Michael had had nothing to eat, but the dancing was something not to be missed, so he grabbed the little piece of roll I had left and we ran out to the waiting car.

The dance had already begun, so we waited for a minute until the music stopped, peering over the heads of the crowd of children and men around the low door. The gypsies live in so-called caves, but the whitewashed, brightly lighted room that we presently went into had little resemblance to any cave. It was, however, dug out of the rock. There was a separate alcove for the kitchen, the walls were clean and white and decorated with shining copper skillets and pans that hung from nails, and with wooden shelves that held more pans and dishes and glasses. The dance stopped and we pushed our way into the room and were cordially led to the far end to two low rush-seated wooden chairs that were placed in the doorway of the bedroom, a smaller but no less spick-and-span cave behind us. There were no gypsy men in the room, only gaily dressed women with long ruffled dresses and hair decorated with combs and flowers. There must have been twenty of them at least, sitting on both sides of the room and taking turns, apparently according to some prede-termined plan, in the various dances and songs. Bottle after bottle of a delicious light dry sherry was consumed both by the dancers and by the audience, the sharp staccato clapping that accompanied the dances like castanets got faster and faster, hair tumbled down in the whirling, cheeks got flushed and the enthusiasm and excitement spread contagiously from dancers to audience until one almost got up to join them. Most of the women dancing that night were relatives of the gypsy Carmen something who is now having such a success in New York.

Poor Michael was again involved with me, but this time he had had enough sherry so that he forgot to worry about what Mrs. Hayes would think, because the gypsies took it for granted that we were married since we came in together and since I was obviously a "nice" girl and nice girls don't go out at that hour unchaperoned except with their husbands. So I was called *Señora* and when they started telling fortunes, one of them hoping for an extra tip told Michael that I would soon have a baby, that it would be a boy and that it would look just like him! At that point we didn't dare disillusion them, so we beamed fatuously at each other and tried to look like a staid married couple. But I later told Michael that since I had known him scarcely twenty-four hours, that was mighty quick work.

It was after two by the time we got home to bed, so we by mutual consent delayed our starting hour the next morning until ten o'clock. The four of us had breakfast together and then agreed to meet for lunch about 2:30 at a little *auberge* run by the government, one of a series that are placed at half-day runs along the main highways. The drive was long and hot and dusty, but Michael was a pleasant companion and we chatted, were silent, chatted again and then I dozed until lunch time.

We got to Madrid about nine o'clock, I left my baggage at the Ritz, powdered my nose, and came right down to the embassy to report in [and tell Father I had arrived]. It was a happy moment for me, as you can imagine. Father was able to get away about ten and we went back to the hotel for a simple "early" supper and then to bed. I was amazed that I was able to sleep at all, I was so excited and everything seemed to me so incredible.

Well, that completes my journey. The next installment will be "Housekeeping and its Problems, particularly in a language one doesn't speak." Perhaps you can give me some pointers on that?

25 July 1944

Dear Father: [probably addressed to New York]

Life continues here its pleasant and unhurried way. I am *en train de* being accepted as a member of the Velasquez Club and have already been there twice as a guest for lunch. I spent all last Sunday walking and exploring the city, by myself, and for the first time feeling a little more relaxed. I had no idea how tired and how tense I was when I came—I feel positively floppy now by comparison. Even sudden noises no longer make me jump as badly, and while fire-crackers in the middle of the night make me wake up with my heart in my mouth, I can now turn over and go to sleep again. In other words I am well on the way to becoming a normal civilian again, a rather comfortable feeling.

Apartment hunting turned out to be such a discouraging procedure that I decided to take that one we looked at on the ground floor. It has so many advantages that I felt the slightly higher rent was justified—electric refrigerator, telephone switchboard, proximity to work, complete absence of dirt and wildlife and the owner's willingness to make whatever changes I wished, within reason of course. I have today taken unto myself a maid, and I hope to move the end of the week. I will try to write you and Mother more about it once I am installed.

In spite of the unreality, it was wonderful to see you again. I hope that next time we meet, it will be on more familiar ground. Chocorua, preferably.

25 July 1944

Dear Mother: [probably addressed to Chocorua]

From here, I am afraid that I cannot adhere to a regular schedule as far as outgoing mail is concerned. Each letter is limited to two pages, so perhaps I shall sometimes write more than once a week, but I will be unable to say that every Monday, for instance, a letter will go to you. But I will do my best to see that some sort of communication goes to you at least once a week.

For some reason, when I first got here I was tense and unaccepting, but suddenly Saturday evening I just seemed to relax and realize what a nice place this might be. And so I went on my first "expotition" [as Christopher Robin called his expeditions] and took my first faltering footsteps in the language. I don't know why it has taken me so long to show any interest and/or initiative in the city—with other new environments I had always been among the first to go exploring and wandering down the little side streets. It was as if for a while I had reached the point of saturation and was unable to accept any new experiences and adventures. But ten days of being inactive and all at once I was eager to get out on my own. Luckily it was Saturday night because I could continue my tour on Sunday. My objective Saturday was to find the best route to the little British embassy chapel, so that I could attend Sunday. But that was merely rationalization and I wandered in and out of narrow streets, window-shopped to my heart's content (fortunately most of the stores were closed and the only purchases I could make were a large straw hat to wear to church the next day and a gay pair of red and white canvas espadrilles), gazed at pushcarts piled with fruits and vegetables, and smiled at all the children playing hopscotch in the streets. It is incredible to me still, and slightly frustrating, to see such a variety of things for sale. I cannot realize that there is no need to rush in and buy something in case one needs it six months from now. And how I wish that I could send some of the things to Buff, both for her personal and for her Red Cross use. Wool, needles, zippers, elastic, raffia, hardware of all sorts, china and glassware, yards and yards of all kinds of material, silver, books—it is just as well I am having this interim period here, can you imagine what effect the window of a Walgreen's drugstore would have on me, directly arrived from North Africa? I wonder how long it will be before I get over my hoarding impulses (which, I must admit, came to me quite naturally).

Madrid, at least in the summer time, is a city of incredibly blue skies and hundreds of darting swallows. I can lie in my bed in the morning and watch them wheel and swoop, when I am taking my siesta they are still there, and in the evening, just before supper, when the sky is most breathtaking and unbelievable blue of all, they are more active and graceful than ever, stuffing themselves most likely on insects that appear after the first heat of the day is gone.

If I had been able to get to Madrid as originally planned, it would have been much better, but during the hot summer months government offices and embassies closed down almost completely and moved to summer quarters in cooler San Sebastian. This explains why my boss was away so much the time and why I felt so discouraged.

7 August 1944

Dear Father and Mother:

I am installed in my new apartment and am very happy there. My maid is proving more than satisfactory and in spite of the language difficulties, we get along together very well and seem to understand more or less intuitively what we are saying to each other. She is a little disappointed, I think, that I eat so little, but she has accepted that now and no longer argues with me.

Physically I am not suffering at all. On other counts I am not too happy. My boss is still away and time hangs very heavy on my hands. For a little while I enjoyed it, but now I am bored to death. . . . In my last job I had so much to do, so much responsibility and the opportunity to be of real use, that this being an inactive second fiddle is very hard. Every once in a while I get "farmed out" and that helps pass the time a bit. . . .

I don't like to start fussing so soon, because I am very glad to be here at last, but I do so badly want a real job that I can get my teeth into, work hard at, get tired over, and have the comfortable feeling at the end of the day that something has been accomplished through one's own efforts and cerebrations. Exploring the city and the vicinity is impossible because whether there is work to do or not, I must be in the office; social life goes on so late at night that I can indulge in it but seldom and anyway I am not much interested, and the result is a pretty empty feeling. While this war lasts, my life is primarily my job, whatever and wherever it is, either Red Cross as it was or State Department as it is, and my personal life and pleasures I have postponed until *dopo la guerra*. It was because I felt that way that I broke my engagement when I came overseas, [and] that even after meeting Doug I went on with my resignation from the Red Cross [which meant moving farther away from him], but darn it all, when one's job doesn't fill one's life and when one has put aside all else, what does one do?

147

In between feeling frustrated, I do have a pretty good time. A new friend took me out to dinner last night, with another chap, and we went out to the former university city of Alcalá de Henares, the birthplace of Cervantes I am told. It was a pleasant drive out, cool after the heat of the day, and the Inn of the Students was very picturesque. The ceilings were high wooden beamed ones, the floor a well-worn flagged one, there was a tremendous fireplace, and the tables were long dark refectory-type with wooden settles. There was a big lantern hung in the middle of the room and the walls were decorated with gay saddle blankets, braided halters, big ladles and such things. In one corner of the room was a stone jug as high as I am, which used to be filled with water or oil. A scene from *If I Were King* could have been played there, someone should have been playing on a guitar, the waitresses should have been pink-cheeked and gaily dressed and humming songs as they passed the wine of the house. It was just like going back a couple of hundred years. The little courtyard with the fig tree growing in the middle was dark and dimly lit as we came through, the stone drinking trough beside the well, the sides of which were grooved by centuries of having the bucket chain sliding up and down. After supper we went into one of the old lecture halls, with a wonderfully carved ceiling and lists of students on the walls, including Ignatius de Loyola, and the garden, surrounded by shadowed cloisters, was just taking the shape of the little formal beds of box and flowers by the light of the full moon which was coming over the top of the tower. Quite incredibly lovely.

On August 10, I wrote a long letter describing my apartment and its contents in great detail, drawing a map of the layout of rooms and the location of some. I concluded:

My maid, Saturia, is really the boss of my household, not me, and I feel continually that I must act in accordance with her wishes and pleasures. She was very upset this morning because I didn't drink a glass of milk before I went to bed. I had one before I went out to dinner and I never thought that she would have another one in the icebox for me. But she did and berated me this morning. And I thought for a few minutes that she would not let me go out at all last night. It is partly your fault, Mother. The trouble was that I had clean white shoes and clean white gloves and was carrying a blue purse! That worried her no end and she almost made me promise to go buy a white one today! Apparently she used to be a lady's maid for some duchess or something and she loves to fuss over little things like that. That was why she was not happy with her previous employer as that was a masculine household and she was only the second maid or something. Now she runs the apartment and the cooking and me, and she is *muy contenta*, and so am I. Whenever I make any purchases, half the fun comes in showing them to Saturia and she gasps and admires and says "*magnifico*" in a very satisfactory manner.

I wrote again the next day, primarily to apologize for the "fussing" I had done, then added:

I broke into the upper brackets last night and had dinner with Mrs. Hayes [wife of the ambassador, who was a friend of Father's] and Mary Elizabeth [Hayes], Findley Burns and some others before the movie in the embassy garden. It was most pleasant—cocktails first in the garden, then a delicious supper on the terrace—with even corn on the cob, an item which was most disappointing to all of us as apparently they gave Mrs. Hayes corn that was almost in the popping class, sort of hard on the outside like dried corn, and while it looked simply beautiful, it was much too hard to eat. (We guests pretended to enjoy this special treat, not daring to put the ears of corn aside until after Mrs. Hayes had tried to eat hers. She quickly declared them inedible and with great relief we were able to relax our diplomatically courteous pretense and enjoy the rest of the meal.) Then peaches and ice cream for dessert and coffee in the garden again. I enjoy Mrs. Hayes very much—she wanted to know if I had heard from you and if you were home, to which I replied in the affirmative and she remarked that you must have seen the ambassador, but nary a word did she say about the note I wrote her and about your offer to carry a message for her. Very strange. Mary Elizabeth seems a nice girl and I think I shall invite her to my housewarming when and if I have one. If I don't spend all my money on other things, I mean. I adore the garden here at the embassy and it is such a nice feeling to have dinner with even part of a family. I get awfully tired of just my own age, and all these on the surface parties. The embassy, even though it is rented, seems more like a home and it is nice to have two generations.

14 August 1944

Dear Mother and Father:

Becky and I (no, Becky is no one that either of you know. She has the apartment next to mine) left about 10:30 Sunday morning and went down by streetcar. It is the first time that I have ridden in a public conveyance since I left home! Streetcars here are lots of fun, because you can stand on the platform and window-shop as you go along. They are never in a hurry and go so slowly that you can really see everything in the store windows without any trouble. And they go down lots of little streets that otherwise you might never explore. A very satisfactory means of transportation, I think. We went almost all around the Plaza Mayor, as most good streetcars do, it being sort of the central meeting place of all streetcars, with a veritable maze of tracks leading in all directions in and out of the gates at the four corners. The Plaza Mayor is a big square completely enclosed by wide arcades topped with three-story buildings. The arcades do not have as elegant shops as those on the Rue de Rivoli, but the impression is much the same. Each long roof is divided in three parts by two slender spires that reach their weather vane and gilded cross high into the blue sky. Close to the arcades run the trolley tracks, leading in and out of the eight arched gates, one at each end of the arcade, and in the middle of the Plaza is a big oval paved promenade, with fountains playing, children running about, grownups resting on the stone benches and the customary equestrian statue in the very middle.

We got off the streetcar outside a big open-air market, which reminded me a little of the one in Constantine where last summer I used to buy precious tomatoes and fresh fruits and vegetables. Heaped on the curb was a tremendous pile of yellow melons, pushcarts were being piled with them for peddling through the streets. In the next square preparations were being made for a fiesta. A carousel was being set up, shooting galleries were under construction, ice cream booths being decorated and there was a general hustle and bustle and air of gaiety that was very contagious. Just beyond all this hubbub was a black sea of people with occasional bright-colored awnings sticking up above their heads. For blocks and blocks, down a steep street and up another one, in and out of alleys stretched the wares of the *Rastro* [Thieves' Market]. I have never seen such a sight, so much junk and so many people. Sometimes it was a real shop on the street that had opened its doors for the Sunday trade, sometimes it was a booth built on the sidewalk, sometimes it was just a display of wares right on the sidewalk and/or street itself—and sometimes it was all three or four so that in order to see everything one would have to make four trips up and down the aisles. Everything in the world, or at least in Spain, eventually finds its way to the *Rastro*, I think. There isn't anything you could name that wasn't there.

In front of one display a brown gypsy woman (*gitana*) squatted on her haunches, a lovely brown baby in her arms, while she bargained over the price of a meter of checked gingham. Some of the gypsies are most unattractive, but every once in a while you will see a beautiful one, like this one, the traditional spit curl of dark hair pasted on her brown cheek. One day in downtown Madrid I saw an older gypsy walking along unconcernedly, although everyone was turning around to stare. She had on white knit stockings with a pattern down the sides (and her legs were far from slender), a long full skirt that came to halfway below her knees and was full enough so that it gave the feeling that there were at least four other skirts beneath it, a large flowered shawl crossed on her chest and a black scarf over her head and tied under her chin. Her face was lovely too, old and brown and wrinkled and very placid. I don't think she even noticed the stares of the passers-by.

Further down the hill and past the square with the church, were all the odds and ends, the notions, the china, the hardware and the plain junk with old broken chamber pots, faded oil paintings, hundreds of rusty screws, an old violin with all the strings gone, all mixed together. I was afraid that my love of buying things would result in my going slightly berserk with so much around me, but there was too much and it was impossible to concentrate on any one thing long enough to buy it. And then best of all, I bought two small triangular black lace *mantillas*, very lovely ones and not too expensive. Saturday evening I bought a fan painted with Spanish scenes, so now I am all fixed and can go native in the best way. I have been wanting to go into some of the churches here, but I have only one hat and that a large conspicuous one, and here everyone wears *mantillas* to church, never hats. Now I have my own *mantilla* and can go without causing comment! In Rome, you know.

After over two hours of pushing our way through the crowds and being "bumped" into and pushed back at every step, Becky and I were ready to quit. So we found a quiet bar and refreshed ourselves with a glass of cold beer, and came home for lunch. Saturia (I have just found that that is the correct spelling) was much pleased with my purchases and showed me the right way to wear the *mantilla*. Oh, I forgot to tell you that at her insistence I finally bought a white pocketbook on Saturday, so that when I went out Saturday night I met with her full approval. Awful, the way my maid pushes me around! She firmly showed me some meringues she bought for Sunday lunch telling me that since I was having a *Señorita* for lunch it would not be polite for her to indulge in my foolish notion of just fruit for dessert!

18 August 1944

Dear Mother and Father:

Isn't the war news wonderful? [The invasion of southern France—code name Anvil—had occurred; much of what we were doing in Algiers was preparing for this.] I am much more excited about this second landing than I ever was over the first, and I am learning to read Spanish in spite of myself, just because I cannot bear to not understand the morning paper. It is only natural, I suppose, that this landing should seem more of a personal thing to me, because I am sure I know so many of the people who participated in it and who have been working for it for so long. It makes me more restless and discontented than ever, to be sitting here in this luxurious idleness while real work is going on elsewhere. I even regret a bit that I left my last job, because letters from there indicate the pressure of work is as great as ever and they are still working twelve to fourteen hours a day, seven days a week. And here I sit, reading all my boss's books and knitting my sweaters. Peg assures me that when (or perhaps I should say if) he returns next week, things will be quite different. I hope so, but I still feel that there is no need for two girls in this office, and that with a few changes and a more efficient schedule one girl could handle it all without too much trouble. Peg is going away for a long weekend as soon as he comes back, so I shall have a bit of a chance to prove my theories, at least for my own satisfaction. Of course, I might quite easily be wrong. I often am.

My social schedule has expanded to include badminton in the embassy garden twice a week. One day last week when I was sitting out by the porter's lodge waiting for Bill to pick me up for lunch at the Club, Mary Elizabeth [the ambassador's daughter] came by and I showed her the *mantillas* I had bought at the Thieves' Market. She, of course, admired them and then wanted to know if I played badminton. I told her I had, several times in my youth, but that I wasn't very good. She said she wasn't either and would I join them the following evening. I did so, in fear and trembling, expecting that they would all be experts. There are six of us, Mary Elizabeth, Mrs. Baldwin, Jim Ford from the naval attaché's office, Larry Spilman, an air attaché, and Colonel Ebright from the military attaché's office. The men are much better than the girls, but no one is expert and we all giggle about it and have a wonderful time.

Life is further complicated these days by Tuesdays, Thursdays and Sundays being without electricity from early in the morning until nine at night. It is things like that that make me glad I live on the ground floor and don't have to walk up countless flights of stairs on the days the elevators don't work. The only inconvenience at my house is that the refrigerator is electric, but we find that the coolness lasts over that period sufficiently.

Walking to the Club the other noon, it occurred to me again how much one would miss if one had no sense of smell. There was the smell of leather and shoe polish as I went by a cobbler's, the sweetness of perfume from a drugstore, a restaurant gave out a strong odor of garlic, a bakery that of fresh-baked cakes, oranges from a fruit store, salt and fish from a fish store, beer from the corner bar and, best of all, the clean smell of pine wood from the little space between two houses where one could buy charcoal and junky pieces of pine for the kitchen stove. And I remember all the smells, nice and otherwise, that I used to delight in last summer walking down a hot street in Constantine. Spices particularly. Here in Madrid there are the extra smells of streets being watered in the sun, the smell of wet earth when the garden is being hosed, the week when all the trees along the streets were in bloom and gave forth a strange sweetness of their own, and the smell of the wood being burned in the Madrid taxis. It is required here, apparently, that all taxis be as old as possible, with wheels that threaten to come off and upholstering that comes apart and seats that sag. An old, old man usually drives, with a child of ten or younger on the seat beside him to help if necessary. No car starts unless it is first vigorously cranked and even so the least little hill will make it stop immediately. Every five blocks or so, hill or not, it stops anyway, and then the child jumps down, runs around back, and stirs up the fire in the sort of boiler that sits on the back fender. Tremendous clouds of smoke and sparks are the result of this stirring, but usually no motion. Then the old man hobbles around, puts on a new piece of wood, says the magic words, stirs the fire again—both he and the little boy disappear at this point behind the clouds—then they hasten around front, crank the taxi again and jump aboard to pull all the levers and pulls possible. Then sometimes it marches. And sometimes it doesn't, in which case the procedure is repeated. If it is repeated five times with no results, you are then allowed to get another taxi—if you can find one! Jeeps may have been more windy and more bouncy, but they were certainly more trustworthy and a better means of transportation. That is, if you really have to get anywhere at any particular time, which seems to be largely an American bad habit. The Spanish really don't care. And I am learning fast.

21 August 1944

Dear Mother and Father:

Oh, what a lovely day I had yesterday. Vinnie (who is my most constant escort as his wife's name is Elizabeth and he calls her Lee, so it makes him feel at home to be with me!)— anyway, Vinnie and I went to Toledo (*not* Ohio).

We took a 9:15 train in the morning, and I think if the day had been nothing but a train ride, I would have been just as excited. The last time I was on a train was that dismal ride from Albany to New York after my visit to Bob's [my then-fiancé] cousin, about twenty months ago. And I haven't been on a continental train since 1936 when I took the boat train from Paris. Any trains are fun but continental ones are really thrilling. As a result of all my movie going and book reading, I expect them to be crowded with international spies, Simon Templar, Jonah and Berry, *The Lady Vanishes*, Marlene Dietrich and many others. As a result, from the moment we stepped into the dirty station with its smoky sooty smell and the noise of train whistles and puffing engines making it almost impossible to talk and the crowds of Sunday travelers impeding one's progress, I was in a perfect lather of excitement and I felt as if my eyes were as big and round as saucers in my attempt to see everything and everybody at once. The only thing that spoiled it was the compartments did not open directly onto the platform; as in American trains one had to get on at the end of the car. But there was the usual side corridor, down which one can wander casually in order to peer into all the other compartments to make sure that Moriarty [Sherlock Holmes's archenemy] wasn't there, and we fortunately had seats on the corridor side so that it was easy to watch the activities of the other members of our compartment by looking in the glass beside one. It was, however, a very dull trip and I didn't see even one person who looked like a jewel thief, except maybe the rather large man who sat across from me with a buxom "blonde" who was obviously not his wife. But we kept meeting them all day doing the usual sightseeing, so I am afraid even he was just a harmless tourist. I hope I have better luck next time!

The station at Toledo was a magnificent more-or-less modern structure (modern in time not design), and Vinnie and I took our time in leaving the train, letting the others knock each other down in a mad rush for the *autobus* which would take them to the town itself. I was wearing my new blue green linen dress which I had made here (very pretty indeed), low-heeled rubber-soled sandals, and carrying a large straw basket with our cameras, films, my *mantilla* to cover my head when we visited the numerous churches—and to hold all the purchases we knew we would make.

The walk to the town was fascinating and I felt sorry for the *autobus* people who missed all that we saw. Outside the station gates was a small collection of one-story whitewashed houses, a couple of cafés and a sort of an inn. There were several beautiful yokes of oxen in the street and a lean greyhound beside them. I wish I had taken a picture of that, but we didn't stop. Down the road a piece was a small caravan of gypsies with their covered carts and the usual accompanying children and dogs. Through the archway leading to the courtyard of the inn we could see horses tethered to the wall, another greyhound, a woman washing clothes at the fountain and a baby playing in the dust. Then around a curve of the road, there was the muddy river Tagus below us to the right with green fields out beyond it on the other bank and rising up in front of us, on the hilltop, the rooftops and church spires of Toledo. We crossed the river on the "towered and turreted medieval bridge of Alcantara," stopping to watch a funeral procession go by, the two horses tossing the white plumes on their heads, the glass-sided Cinderella coach with the white coffin inside (white is for a child), and the solemn group of mourners on foot behind.

Then we toiled up the steep steps, instead of going around more gradually by the road, to the top of the hill and to the town itself. We had turned down various offers from guides, and for an hour or more we just wandered as our fancy dictated, up and down narrow cobbled streets, into sunny squares and through shady archways, peeking into open doors through which one could see the inner courtyard and gardens, hanging plants, latticed windows and little fountains that reminded me so much of the Arab and Moorish houses I had seen in North Africa. As it was Sunday morning, the

157

church bells were ringing in various parts of the town and we met little groups of women hurrying up the streets, black lace scarves over their heads and fans and prayers books in their hands. A little bent old man in a gray smock showed us through the Museo de San Vicente, which used to be a church and now holds an incredible collection of church robes, tapestries, silver and gold and coral chalices and El Greco paintings.

I consulted the Baedeker again and we went down the hill a bit to the ruined chapel of Santa Cristo de la Luz which has a nice story attached to it, which I will tell you sometime when I have more space. It used to be a mosque. The care-taker took us through his garden in back and up on top of the Puerta del Sol, the old main gate to the city. The top is crenelated, and much of the old part has been restored—it gives a magnificent view of the entire city and the valley around it. (Maybe, Father, your picture book of Spain will show some pictures of the things I mention here.) From the gate we went back up to the main square, called the *Zocodover,* which used to be the centre of the Moorish *souks* or markets. We shopped a bit for Toledo steel souvenirs. Later in the afternoon, we went into one of the workshops and watched them do some of the work. It is amazingly beautiful—some of the swords can be bent into a perfect circle.

On the way to the cathedral we were picked up by a per-sistent guide who finally got possession of my basket and refused to leave us. We gave in at last and were much amused by his tales and the way, after we paid him at the end, in which he asked for a cigarette and the gleam in his eye as he tucked it behind his ear and swaggered off down the street. We took a lot of pictures, my favorite one being of a pure white cat drinking from a fountain in front of the cathedral. I don't know when I can send the pictures to you, both those we took and the millions of cards I bought, but I shall investigate and send them with notations as soon as I can. The rest of the afternoon was more conventional. We went to Santo Tomé which has an El Greco in it, then down to a fourteenth-century synagogue, then to El Greco's house and museum, back up and through the cathedral, more postcards, more shops, to the cafe again, and then a leisurely wandering down the hill to the bridge, back to the station with time out for a beer at the cafe across the street and the excitement of seeing a tremendous bull being led up the street, and the train ride back to Madrid.

The day ended hilariously by the train being held up or breaking down or something about a quarter of a mile outside the station, this happening just as the heavens opened and the long-awaited and wanted rain came down. We sat for over half an hour and then got bored, so jumped out on the tracks and ran through the rain [and] through the dark to the station. It was a little scary because there were so many tracks and trains could come from both directions, but we made it, walked dripping through the station just as our train pulled in after all, took a taxi home to wash, and then down to a little Spanish restaurant for supper. The supper itself wasn't too unusual, but for dessert we had a huge dish of fresh strawberries from Valencia, the most ambrosial thing I have eaten for years. By this time we were both so sleepy that we weren't even talking, we taxied home, I took a bath and washed my hair (since it was so wet anyway) with my eyes shut, and fell into bed. It was nice and cool, the rain was still coming down and I was asleep almost before I hit the pillow.

28 August 1944

Dear Mother and Father:

Well, life is really on the upswing again and I am happy at last. Peg left Saturday on a ten-day vacation and the Boss and I are working like mad and having a wonderful time. I got up Saturday morning for the first time since I got here with a yen to go to work, knowing that there would be work and plenty of it. It is a darn nice feeling. Yes, I know I am crazy—but then I inherited it from you. The office is a combination of a lunatic asylum and Grand Central Station in ten different languages, and I love it. Today has been just as nice, and I rushed home late for lunch and rushed back here, knowing that this would be the only time I would have to write you. You'd better appreciate it.

Sunday I had been invited some time ago to go out to the country with the Baldwins. Anyway, I asked the Boss if he intended to work Sunday, and he said that he might come in for a piece but that my services would not be needed. So with a clear conscience I departed the city about 10:30. I have been trying to find on the map the name of the place where we went, but it doesn't seem to be shown. It is not far from Avila, along the river that comes down near there. The drive out was beautiful, about two hours it took, first through yellow plains, through villages of stone cottages with bunches of figs hanging drying in the sun beside the door and children and dogs playing together in the cobblestone streets, then into the bare and rocky hills and finally into the pine forest along the river. The sky was a brilliant blue with wind-whipped clouds piled high on the horizon, magpies flashed up from the road in front of us and swallows dipped over the stubbled fields. The low green vines in the vineyards along the road hung heavy with clusters of purple grapes, haystacks shone in the sun and the wind lifted sudden clouds of chaff from the beaten-down circle where during the week they flail out the wheat. Then the incredible greenness of the pine trees and the nostalgic aroma from the thick bed of needles on the ground and the song of the wind in the branches . . . To be in the country again was wonderful, I felt like a feather in comparison to the dull leaden feeling I have had for so long. We crossed the river as it came through a notch in the hills (I cannot really call them mountains) and met it again further up where it had been dammed in order to utilize the water for the electricity in Madrid. When one saw how pathetically low the water was in the reservoir, with the shelved sandy mudbanks dry and white like bones long in the sun, one no longer wonders at the three (and threatened four) currentless days we now have. But the water that was left was heavenly cool—our dressing room was a pine-covered hill the sides of which were crisscrossed with goat paths—and we swam for almost two hours.

[After lunch] . . . we swam again and sat on another rock and talked some more, then got dressed and had "tea," another watermelon, and drove leisurely home. I was sunburned and weary and sleepy and very happy. And very grateful to the Baldwins for one of the nicest days I have had since I have been here.

Siesta time is up and the Boss is back. So I must stop. He sends his love to all of you and says he really will write you soon.

1 September 1944

Dear Mother and Father:

Boy, what a rest cure this is turning out to be! It makes my previous job seem like that of an amateur. Not only are the hours longer at times, but the pressure is terrific, with an average of three or so deadlines a day. Down yonder we worked hard, but only twice a week did things have to be done at a certain time, so there was more leeway about doing them. In other words, if you typed up something tonight or tomorrow morning did not make much difference. Here I am in such a rush that I even fell down the backstairs of the embassy yesterday! Just shook me up a bit and I am quite black and blue, but it just goes to show. Monday, when I wrote you last, I worked top speed from 9 A.M. to 2:15, back at 3 to write you but even that got cut short, and then straight through with not a break until 11 that night! I love the working hard, but I wish one could eat about 8 and then come back to work. Waiting until 11 makes me even more tired and then I am too tired to eat much when I do get

161

home. But it is fun, and I shall be sorry when Peggy comes back. The Boss is fun to work with and for, but very distracting. Nothing is ever done in sequence. I will be typing a report and he will interrupt to read me something or ask me a question or dictate a letter or want to send a cable, or else the telephone will ring or someone knock on the door. Very hectic and confusing and if I have anything long and requiring concentration, the only way to do it is to get him out of the office.

By the way, he says he is very hurt that not even regards were sent to him in either letter from you received yesterday! Joan's was the only one that mentioned him at all.

When he was in a low mood the other day, I pulled out that wonderful picture of you, Father, smelling the flowers! It cheered him up at once and he now has it on the desk in front of him. He also says he is hurt that a copy was not sent to him. So I don't know whether I shall ever get it back or not. [I still have it, so he *did* give it back.]

The ambassador was not here long enough for me to pay my respects to him. I shall when he returns from the seashore. Nice of him to be so cordial to you about it.

I had a nice but rather blue letter from the girl who took my place [in Algiers]. She is doing almost the entire job single-handed.

I spent one of the most delightful evenings I have had since I got here last night. Tom Bowie had a small party at his apartment and invited me. I went with Keeler Faus, who was interned with Paul duVivier, and also there was David something who played the fiddle at the square dance and his French wife and his colleague in relief work here named Larry something. (I am feeling very old today. Tom's birthday is today and I found out that he is only just 27, and I had thought he was at least three years older than me.) We didn't do anything exciting. Keeler brought two recorders with him and those were played, David had his violin, Tom plays a cornet, and there was a piano which we played both

162

with and without the player attachment. It was most amusing to see Tom sitting at the piano, music coming forth and him playing the cornet at the same time. We sang a bit and talked a lot, had a delicious dinner during which we argued long and loud about Paris being the center of the fashion world and whether it would be after the war or not, and in general had the sort of pleasant evening at home that one finds here so seldom. Keeler and I are going bookstall shopping on Sunday morning, I think, and Tom has asked me to come back and practice on the piano so that there can be a piano accompaniment the next time we sing, and I am quite happy about the whole thing. But I still don't like Madrid!

I don't think I told you about the time I impressed even myself. I was walking along the street, going to work one afternoon, looking very *tipica* in espadrilles and carrying a straw basket, and just as I was passing a little fruit store down the street, one of the C.D. *[Corps Diplomatique]* cars drives past. A big one, complete with uniformed chauffeur etc. There is a man inside the fruit store buying some fruit. He kind of glances at me as I pass, then there is this grinding of brakes and squealing of tires as the big car comes to a sudden stop, the chauffeur having recognized me. He, the chauffeur, leaps out to open the door for me, the man in the store almost falls into a basket of peaches as I nod graciously at the chauffeur and get into the car. We drive off in style, leaving the man in the store gaping after me. Fun.

Well, again the siesta is almost up and I have four thousand things to do this afternoon. Have a feeling this is going to be another one of those days. However, I shall not fall down the back stairs today, as I am now brazenly using the front marble ones—the entire family being away.

[Undated]

Dear Mother and Father:

I might just as well begin at the beginning. Friday, as I anticipated, was quite a day. Another until-eleven-o'clock one, but very satisfying and my week's work here has earned me some nice compliments from the Boss who says something about my being most competent and capable of accepting much responsibility. (I repeat this just for your benefit, not of course, that I derive any pleasure!) He later said however that I was the hardest girl he had ever worked for! Saturday was another long day, but I did manage to get my two hours at lunch time and go to the Club.

Sunday I had the whole day off again, which was an unexpected luxury. Findley and I went to early service at the British church (I felt very *tipica* in my black lace scarf), then I came home to breakfast and fussed around the house for an hour or so, and then Keeler came to take me shopping at the bookstalls down at the end of the Retiro. I knew that would be fun, but it was much more so than I had anticipated. There are about thirty stalls lined up with their backs to the fence of the park, and in a little over two hours we covered only twelve of them! Books have always been one of my loves, and apparently Keeler is as fond of them as I am. He has boxes and boxes of them waiting for him in Paris [where he had been stationed as a foreign service officer], and when I saw the numerous items of baggage he has in his apartment, I felt a little less badly about my own acquisitive instincts and habits. I have a feeling that going shopping with him is going to have very bad effects on both of us, as we sort of egg on each other.

You have never seen such a collection of books in your life, all kinds, sizes, ages, conditions, languages and subjects. The displays in front were more for the taste of the casual buyer, while in back were shelves and shelves for the more serious book collector. I doubt very much if there was anything really valuable, but there was plenty that was interesting. The subjects ranged from a pile of thin mid-Victorian (not quite but almost) books on morals for children (Keeler bought the whole pile), *Babbitt* in French (which I bought), the whole Tom Swift series in English, *Tarzan* in Spanish, a book on fluid dynamics in English, one on beet sugar in

English, Goethe's poems in German, *Medicine in the Home* in Spanish, a wonderful cookbook in French (which I bought), a nice three-volume set of Cervantes (which I bought), Spanish lives of saints, French books on dogs, Conan Doyle's life of David Hume, and down to some shabby copies which looked quite old of à Kempis and others. We were simply entranced and could hardly look at one shelf long enough because the next one looked so interesting. We read titles out loud at the same time, pulled a book off the shelves to look at only to see another one that was more appealing, we bought things right and left, paying a paltry sum for each, and finally about 2:15 we wearily hailed a taxi. My basket was bulging with books, I had a big pile under one arm and a lovely old map and fourteen colored pictures of a bullfight under the other. [The map is now framed and hangs in our Cambridge apartment.] Our hands were filthy, of course, and we even had smudges on our faces from the dust we had raised from books long untouched.

We stopped at my house first and Saturia came running to relieve us of our loads. She was very disapproving of the dirt and said she would dust my books at once and then air them on the window ledge of her room, and then put them in the bookcase. And she told me I must be sure and wash my hands carefully before lunch! So you see I am well taken care of.

Sunday morning after breakfast I wrote you a long letter in shorthand, sort of an *apologia vitae*, trying to put into words why I didn't like it here. But now as I reread it, it doesn't say it the way I hoped it would, so I shall not transcribe it. To say that life here is like food without any seasoning, or like the fluffy part of an ice cream soda, doesn't begin to describe it. There is a superficiality, an aimlessness, a lack of inspiration and common purpose that makes everything seem flat, like stale beer or ginger ale. That is part of it, and another part of it is—nuts, I cannot put it into words. It doesn't matter much, except that I wanted you to know the reason why I am disregarding your recommendation and almost request. It may not do any good, but at least I am trying. Anyway, I don't think I have to explain it to you, because I think you understand how I feel.

Looking back, the "flatness" was due in part to the contrast from the vitality and urgency of the work in Algiers, the letdown after the landing in southern France and the fact that my boss was away so much. All this was compounded by my extreme dislike of having to share the swimming pool at the Club with Germans and Japanese. And also, of course, by the fact that there really wasn't enough work for two secretaries.

A long letter on September 8 about domestic matters ended: "I decided I had been here long enough to suggest some changes in procedure, so I have become a veritable Efficiency Expert, having routing slips printed for incoming correspondence, changing the files and having a lovely time!" Was I perhaps preparing the way to be declared redundant? Mostly in response to a wonderful letter from Father, I wrote again the following day:

Your long keep-your-chin-up letter, Father, was well done and appreciated. I am not sure that my unhappiness here is a matter of conscience, more personal preference as to a way of life. However, if it were not for the war, I might enjoy it a little more—but still not for any length of time. I am gradually reducing the tempo of my life to fit in with the quieter routine here, and I suppose it was the adjustment period that came the hardest. I am more or less (still mostly less) reconciled to it for a while. The appropriate time for the discussion you mentioned has already come up and been taken care of to my complete satisfaction. So now I must again possess my soul in patience, and I must admit that the surroundings are more pleasant here than they were the last time I had to be patient. I am only sorry that my tall friend [my other "title" for the Boss] must be away so much of the time. I

166

have been farmed out during his absence to Kate's husband the apostle. Pleasant and helps pass the time.

I must have discussed my feelings of dissatisfaction with my boss who agreed to set in motion the necessary machinery for my transfer.

The same mail brought a letter from Esther Tyler, my father's secretary, describing the celebration in Rockefeller Plaza of the liberation of Paris, and also one from the Reverend Fr. Whitney Hale, rector of the Church of the Advent in Boston, who had prepared me for baptism and confirmation there a few years earlier. So all in all my mood was ever so much better than it had been for some time. Letters from my parents were always much appreciated, as were the many packages they sent in response to my requests for clothes, toiletries and books; yet letters from non-family members were especially welcome.

12 September 1944

Dear Mother and/or Father:

Even if I had had the time to write you yesterday before the mail closed, I had already used up my allowance of two pages in answering the four letters I got from you on Friday. Hope this Friday does as well.

We were given the use of one of the cars, the we being me and three men! I tried to persuade them that leaving early meant six or at least seven in the morning, but they were adamant and we pulled away from my front door at 8:35. The day was a little overcast but Saturia promised that it would clear up later. We drove out in the direction of Escorial, past it on our left and up the winding road to the pass over the Guadarramas, the Madrid side of the mountains being rocky and fairly barren, but the slopes of the far side covered with pine groves. The view from the top of the pass was wonderful, the sky was getting bluer by the minute and the morning was still pleasantly cool. On the other side of the mountains was a fertile valley, quite a difference from the yellow plain around Madrid, but the valley doesn't extend very far and soon, over another rise of hills, the familiar tawny fields stretch out filled with tremendous granite boulders, split and tumbled into fantastic shapes and piles. We passed through little villages, built close into the fold of a valley so that one was almost through them before one was really aware that they were there. The villages in this part of Spain are much like those in North Africa, the houses close together, the roofs going every which way, the narrow little side alleys of packed dirt (or mud, depending on the season), and the innumerable children, dogs, cats and chickens. I suppose there is not so much an actual similarity as there is an atmosphere that they have in common. Here the roofs are of baked red tiles and the walls so much a part of the earth around them that I cannot remember whether they are grayish yellow or brownish gray. There are no trees but every once in a while there is a tangle of scrub pines and underbrush from which a giant jackrabbit sometimes leaps, or out of which a covey of quail may be flushed. And the big magpies flashed black and white across the road.

Avila of the crenelated walls and towers looks like a storybook picture of a medieval town. It is almost unbelievable and I wouldn't have been at all surprised if knights on horseback had ridden out of one of the imposing gateways and if lovely ladies had leaned down from one of the towers and waved their white handkerchiefs at the lords going off to the tourney or to the wars. I had expected an austere and forbidding city, but it is gay and interesting and just like a fairy tale. We drove past it as Salamanca was first on our list, but we got back about 5:30, just as the light was best, throwing long shadows of one crenelated tower sharply against the crenelated wall just beyond.

The cathedral is more like a fortress, with heavy towers and thick doors, but the inside in tremendous contrast is dim and lofty, cool and lovely. By far the nicest church I have

168

been in since I have been here. I hid behind each pillar, for although my arms were modestly covered with my jacket, my legs were bare and a new edict has recently been put into effect, that dresses must be a certain length and legs must be covered with stockings and sleeves must be long, as well as the head covered—mine most appropriately with my *mantilla*. We went out the back door of the cathedral, which brought us outside the city walls, and walked down to the market square which has a gateway into the city on one side, a row of arcaded buildings on another with cafes underneath, and a lovely little old church on the third. We stopped in the church for a minute and got there just in time for the end of a christening. Around the church, through the little square in back and down the hill, waiting for a minute to let a herd of bulls and cows cross the road, followed by a fat pink and gray pig. I have never seen pigs like that anywhere before. Most of them are a most unattractive shade of dead gray, but once in a while you get a mottled or half and half effect of bright pink and dead gray. Most peculiar.

Speaking of pigs reminds me of the herd of them that we passed just before we came to Avila, driven by a stout and perspiring prioress, her long and voluminous black skirts around her ankles and a willow switch in her hand. The paths along the edge of the road were crowded with people going to the city, for there was a *feria* [festival or fair] and goats, sheep, cattle and pigs were all being taken to market. Children in their Sunday best were perched up behind Father on the back of the family horse, while Mother sat sideways on a burro. Someone should do another Chaucer's *Canterbury Tales* of the Spanish going to a *feria*.

We visited the church attached to the Dominican monastery founded by Ferdinand and Isabella, walked up the hill again past a little church with a tremendous stork's nest on top, the only one I have seen in Spain, along the prome-nade outside the walls, through the gate of St. Theresa, looked into the church which is built on the foundations of the house in which she was born, up through the little Plaza Mayor and past a small vegetable market back to the Cathedral Square. We had noticed earlier the swarming of the cattle *feria* in the valley, so we drove down to see it at first hand and Joe and I walked out into the middle of a field just teeming with bulls and cows that approached you from every angle. I wasn't really scared, but those big black bulls are mighty big and I wasn't comfortable with my back towards one of them. If you know what I mean. I took a couple of pictures that ought to be wonderful if they come out. Just a few minutes before sunset we started back and got to the top of the pass as the last bit of color faded from the sky. And back to Madrid in time for a not-too-late supper.

To go back a bit, we got to Salamanca about 11:30. I was a little disappointed because my guide book had been full of praises of it as a most picturesque and lovely city. To my mind, both Toledo and Avila are better. The two cathedrals, the old and the new, are interesting but the most fun of all was when we climbed up to the spire on one of the towers. The first part of the stairs are very ordinary stairs, then suddenly you come into a living-room-kitchen with a bedroom off it and a balcony in front where the family of the bell ringer lives, I guess. There was a baby on the floor playing with two cats who in turn were playing with some rather old fish. A bit unexpected and startling. Then on up some wooden stairs that in spite of their age seemed very solid, and so into the bell loft. Up past the big bells, on the narrowest, circular stone staircase that I have ever seen. One stair was even worn right through, and all the stairs were covered with sand which made them slippery. With the memory of my falling down the embassy stairs still quite fresh, I wasn't too happy. But the view from the top was magnificent and well worth the climb, the shortness of breath and the uncertainty. A rich green valley with a river winding through it on one side, and the uneven tile roofs of the town on the other three, the roofs often broken by an inner patio or court. It was really lovely and I hope that some of my pictures come out.

We explored part of the old university, walked around the beautiful Plaza Mayor and stopped for a drink, and then found a little restaurant for lunch. We had squid in its own ink gravy! And it was good! After lunch we crossed the river to the horse *feria* and Joe and I walked among the horses and colts and burros and mules, patting soft noses and taking pictures. I liked that part of Salamanca almost best. I took a couple of pictures of the horses with the spires and towers of the city rising up above across the river. And then drove back to Avila.

It was a nice, albeit rather breathless Sunday. I prefer Vinnie as a companion for my sightseeing, as he likes to do the same aimless wandering that I do, just going where the inclination leads, taking pictures and satisfying one's curiosity. My main objection to Spain is that there are too many churches! [I wonder if I'd feel that way if I visited Spain today. Probably not, as churches mean much more to me now than they did then, although I attended Sunday services fairly regularly in the Anglican church in Madrid . . . at least when I wasn't away sightseeing.]

18 September 1944

Dear Mother and Father:

The electricity continues to be a problem. Since the powers that be have returned to town [from summer quarters in San Sebastian], the current is on a good deal of the time—probably because they don't like walking upstairs—but it is likely to go off at odd moments. There was a terrific rain and thunderstorm the other night and right in the middle of supper the lights went off. I had asked Saturia to buy candles but she had put it off, so there we were in the dark. She found my flashlight and I remembered where I had a candle packed away, and got it out. The blackout lasted all evening and I finished supper by candlelight, read for a little while and then took my bath and put up my hair also by its flickering light. Reminded me of the good old days in Chocorua. Kind of fun.

This has certainly been a social week. With the Boss away I thought I should anyway make my bow to the ambassador [Carleton Hayes], so I asked Michael to let me know when he was free for a minute. Michael promised to give me twenty-four hours notice so that I could be dressed a little less casually than usual, but then of course one morning, Friday it was, at eleven o'clock, Michael said I had been asked to lunch that day! I had been out late the night before (Vinnie had taken me to a Spanish musical comedy which was quite amusing). So I had to dash home and take a bath and change my dress and tell Saturia that I would not be home for lunch (she was as much excited about it as I was). Then Michael picked me up in the office at 1:30 and deposited me in the Goya Room or something and very shortly Mrs. Hayes and Mary Elizabeth came down. The ambassador arrived shortly with Michael and the five of us had a most delightful time. I enjoyed him tremendously and, as I have said before, I think Mrs. Hayes one of the most gracious and charming of people. Lunch was delicious, coffee was served in the garden, Father was spoken of very warmly, and between the responsibility of being my father's daughter and the thin ice that we sometimes skated on conversationally [because obviously I couldn't talk about the office for security reasons, but also because Ambassador Hayes wasn't at all happy having intelligence people literally on his doorstep], I turned out to be a most amusing and scintillating luncheon guest. I kept them in continual giggles describing some of the so-called hardships of my Red Cross life, particularly the figure I cut as I staggered up the gangplank of the boat to come across. Mary Elizabeth was nice enough to tell me later that her father had said it was one of the most pleasant luncheons he had had in a long time. (Here I go, blowing my own horn again, but you understand it is only for your pleasure.) I am usually quiet in a gathering of that sort and I was amazed at myself, the way I sort of ran on in this amusing fashion. Felt just like a character in a book. If you know what I mean.

Sunday was supposed to be a day of rest. I told Mrs. Sharp I would sit with her at church, but when my alarm went off at quarter to eight, I just turned it off and went back to sleep. Then I had a breakfast date with a couple of the girls and came home about noon to knit and read *The Little Locksmith*. However, after about half an hour the doorbell rang and Bob Whedbee arrived. He stayed for lunch and then we decided to get out into the country. Like a couple of idiots, we set as our goal the mountain town of Cuenca, about a hundred miles away! The drive down was lovely, at one point we went through a cloudburst and little rivers were running over the road and fields alongside were lakes of water and mud. We got to Cuenca about six, and wandered around for a couple of hours until dusk. It is a small city set up in the hills and looks far removed from civilization and modern times, still being a typical city of the Middle Ages. The views are magnificent, there is an old thirteenth-century cathedral, tiny cobblestone streets, more steps than actual street, houses that lean way over the valley far below. I took some pictures and bought some nice postcards, which will go on their way to you soon. We ate a light supper, mostly omelette and beer, at a little restaurant and then started home. We nearly had to walk most of the way, because the temperature register didn't work and didn't show that there was no water in the radiator, so we almost ruined the engine before it became apparent that something was wrong and we stopped at a farmhouse to get a bucket of water. I drove over half the way—which I disliked intensely as it had been over a year since I had driven and I never did like it much at night—because Bob's eyes got so tired. We got home just before two o'clock—I really appreciated my *siesta* today. However, it was well worth doing and Cuenca is one of my favorite towns in Spain. Next to Avila, I think.

Dear Mother and Father:

Let's see if I can come down to earth long enough to write you some sort of a letter. I am absolutely running around in circles, making lists, getting one suitcase packed and then turning it upside down to find something at the bottom and then repacking it in another way. I didn't think that I had been here long enough to really indulge in my acquisitive habits, but it seems that I am "better" than I thought I was, and have added considerably to my possessions in the short time that I have been in Spain. I am having one suitcase crated and shipped home, so about six months from now you may have to get it out of hock at the customs. It is filled with books, linen and china—and a few odd clothes that I felt I might be able to do without. Do, please, read the books and make use of the other things if you feel so inclined. The only point in possessions is the use that is made of them, and it is silly to have a lot of things packed away and not used. One book called *Perfume from Provence,* which I bought at the bookstalls, reminds me a lot of M. André, what with rabbits and gardens and fruit trees. And you will be amused to see the old bound copy of *St. Nicholas* [the children's magazine] that I also found in the bookstalls and which I thought would be fun to add to the others that we have for the delectation of the next generation. Made me quite homesick looking through it last night. The green material is part of a cargo parachute that someone gave me in Italy. I have always meant to have something made out of it, but just never got around to it, and now I am tired of carrying it around. The boys who gave it to me all had table napkins made out of their part of it and pajamas— but I still don't know what I shall use mine for. Any ideas?

The office is lovely and quiet, as the Boss is out. So I had better stop this writing for pleasure and take care of the few p.p.c. [*pour prendre congé*—to take leave of someone] notes that I must write. My next letter to you should at least have a new heading, at least so I hope.

P.S. I'll write you from place to place so you can keep with me mentally anyway!

A note on 20 September gave no clue to the excitement expressed in a rather incoherent letter dated September 25, my last from Madrid. It is frustrating indeed not to be able to fill in the missing bits . . . perhaps it would have helped if I had saved the letters from my parents as they had saved mine to them. I did write that the Boss was due back the next day and it is more than likely that he had put the wheels in motion while he was away wherever he was. Anyway, I was being transferred to London for reassignment! On October 2 I cabled from Lisbon that I was there and en route to seeing my brother Richard. Even from neutral Lisbon, I refrained from indicating where he was stationed.

CHAPTER SIX

Blackouts and Bomb Shelters

———◆———

October 5–November 19, 1944

On October 20 Gen. Douglas MacArthur stepped ashore in the Philippines to reclaim the islands he had left two and a half years before. The Battle for Leyte Gulf began October 23—the biggest sea battle in history and a tremendous victory for the United States; it initiated the liberation of the Philippines.

On November 7 President Roosevelt defeated the Republican candidate, Thomas E. Dewey, to win an unprecedented fourth term in the White House. His new Vice President was Harry S. Truman, formerly a U.S. Senator from Missouri.

On November 8, the U.S. Third Army in France launched a drive to break through German lines and reach the Rhine River; four days later British Lancaster bombers wrecked the German battleship *Tirpitz* in a Norwegian fjord.

My first letter home from London, dated 5 October 1944 and written on notepaper of the Mount Royal Hotel & Restaurant, Marble Arch, London W1, confirmed my safe arrival. Life in wartime England was incredibly different from what I called the "cream-puff" life in Madrid. I wrote home 12 October to say how glad I was to be away not only from "neutrality" but also from diplomatic life, which was "all right in books but when it comes to living it, a bit of a disappointment."

177

In London I marked time—filling in as a typist here and there in OSS offices and waiting for orders. Always an Anglophile, I found it deeply satisfying just to be in England, perhaps especially because it was an England at war. In addition, my brother Richard, an officer in the Army Signal Corps, was stationed nearby, and a number of family friends were living in or near London, or passing through. Among them were Lewis Gannett, on assignment for the *New York Herald Tribune;* Jessie Aiken Armstrong, whose first husband was the poet Conrad Aiken; and, most especially, Allen Dulles whom I had identified in my letters as "Clover's husband." From Algiers in May I had asked Father almost facetiously if he thought there was a chance that his long-time friend might need a secretary; he did, and I had then expected to go work for him in Switzerland. By the time I arrived in London, the job situation had changed once again and I was not to go on to Berne as planned. Within ten days, however, it all changed again and I had to cable home on 14 October to ignore the previous day's letter.

Finally on 17 October I was able to settle down sufficiently to write one of my narrative letters, bringing my parents up to date on the events of the past month, including my last days in Madrid and the trip to London:

London, England

Dear Mother and Father:

I don't know how much longer I shall be here, just long enough to get the necessary authorizations and so forth. Clover's husband is to be my new boss—do I detect paternal influence there? I am both pleased and sorry. Pleased because it should be most interesting and pleasant, much more so than my last post; sorry because I really did want to finish the war out in a country that was fighting. I like Army people, like having them around and I shall miss them as I did before. Oh well, at least I am out of the country that I disliked so much. I am also sorry to be leaving here. . . . I imagine my new assignment pleases both of you, less to worry about there than here.

I don't think that my letters to you have included my getting out of Spain, have they? The wonderful lunch that our tall friend gave me out at *El Meson,* a sort of inn about ten miles out of Madrid. Bill and Scott were along too, and we ate out on the terrace, looking across the brown plains to Madrid in the distance. There was a flock of sheep grazing below the terrace and the bells around their necks sounded softly in the still air as they lazily moved from one clump of grass to another. An awning over us kept the sun from shining too warmly and we stayed for over two hours, eating and talking and just sitting. Wonderful sherry and olives and pickles and sausage *de la maison,* then Bill and I had partridge done in a casserole with little potatoes and vegetables, delicious bread (unusual in Spain), a good wine, very cold melon for dessert, coffee and a liqueur. And then both Bill and our tall friend bought me some of the pottery that the inn sells, as I remember it was four ashtrays and a sugar bowl and cream pitcher. Those are all in the big suitcase that Peg is sending home for me. Hope they get there safely. In addition, Jane and Joan (office colleagues) each gave a party for me, and Mrs. Hayes (the ambassador's wife) had me to tea. All very pleasant and heartwarming.

The trip to Lisbon was fairly routine. I went all the way there with a clerk from one of the consulates named Lee. . . . The most exciting thing about it was that it was the first time that I had ever flown in a commercial plane. I was amazed at the comfort and convenience. Quite different from the bucket seats that I am accustomed to. We had lovely weather and flew low enough so that I could see much of the country. The first view of Lisbon with the broad and muddy expanses of the Tagus below one is quite something.

After checking in at the hotel, we set out to explore. Both

of us agreed that Lisbon was a big improvement on Madrid, cleaner and less oppressive. We walked for over an hour and then ended up at the harbor and finding a little ferryboat just about to set off, we climbed aboard, first buying a pocketful of hot chestnuts and some cookies from a vendor on the dock. The ride was all too short, just across the river, but we stayed almost a quarter of an hour on the opposite side and when we came back the sun was just setting over the Atlantic at the mouth of the river and the sky there was pink and gold and lavender, and in the other direction a big yellow moon had risen and was bright in the dark eastern sky. In between, the river was quiet and the fishing boats were coming into harbor, with colored sails and patches like the ones we used to see at Les Sables d'Olonnes [which I had visited as a child the summer my father was in Paris working on the Kellogg-Briand Pact]. Some of the bigger boats had high carved prows, and at the mouth of the river were two three-masted sailing ships. It was one of the most beautiful things I have ever seen, there was a gentle breeze welcome after the heat of the day, the other people on the ferry were laughing and gay, the chestnuts were still warm in my pocket, and life was indeed very good. I felt more at peace with myself and happier than I had since I left Algiers. Until I left it [Spain], even though I knew I didn't like the country, I had no idea how oppressive it really was, with sort of an undercurrent of the *Falange* [the fascist organization established in 1934 that helped overthrow the Republic in the Spanish Civil War and became the only official political party during Franco's regime] and what they stood for that permeated every corner of life there.

We ate once in a bullfighter's restaurant, went out to Estoril for dinner at the Casino where there was supposed to be dinner dancing, and as soon as we finished our soup and the music started, Lee and I made for the dance floor, to get there before the crowd. We did all right, for the crowd never came! Apparently in Portugal they are more interested in eating than dancing and no one danced until dinner was over. We stood it for two dances, solemnly revolving around alone on the big dance floor, with everyone in the place almost falling out of their chairs to watch us, and then we could take it no longer and retreated to our table. It really was amusing, but a little conspicuous.

And then there was the family of Germans who lived in the same hotel with us. Papa who was very Prussian and stiff like a poker, Mama who was round and shapeless and very much the *hausfrau*, two daughters about 16 and 14 with long blond braids to below their waists, and expressionless faces, and then the little daughter, aged about six, with blond hair cut Dutch fashion. Every meal they ate way at the back of the dining room, and every meal they left in exactly the same fashion. First came the six-year-old to open the door and close behind came the oldest daughter, carrying a bottle of table water in one hand and an apple or a bunch of grapes in the other. Two minutes later came the second daughter, also with a bottle of table water and carrying either fruit or three or four rolls. Three minutes later came Mama, with both hands full of whatever she could gather from the table. And a good five minutes after all of them, completely ignoring the curious glances of the rest of the dining room, came Papa with a plate full of food and a knife and fork. It was an amazing sight and we could never figure out what they did with the food or why they took it from the dining room. There just seemed to be no logical explanation.

Tuesday morning on the first day flight since the beginning of the war, we left for the U.K. At the airport an English woman came up to me and introduced herself, saying that her young daughter Dinah was traveling with me, going to England to join up, and would I sort of look after her. Dinah was a very pleasant looking girl of just 17 1/2 and I agreed with pleasure. There were only five of us: the British attaché for air, Dinah, Lee, myself and a very large and portly Dutch gentleman, so large that his chair was on one side of the plane and the four of us on the other! The trip wasn't too tedious, we had an excellent box lunch which included a small bottle of port, and although it was very cold, we were not really uncomfortable. I had a slight case of Madrid tummy, the first, which made things a little awkward but that was all. We were well above the clouds, of course, and looking down on them with glimpses of the blue sea below, made one feel that one was flying upside down, looking at the clouds with sky beyond. The Scilly Isles looked very tiny and England incredibly neat and trim. Customs and security took an awfully long time but finally we were cleared and the bus took us to the hotel in Bristol. [There was a problem with my diary which for some reason they wanted to confiscate. Eventually I persuaded them to let me keep it. Otherwise this letter could never have been written!] My first impression was that of warm friendliness, and eagerness to do everything they could to make us comfortable and happy. A very nice welcome. Dinah and I shared a room, and after supper the three of us took a long walk around the dark town. Dinah had not been in England since the war and she was wide-eyed over the damage done.

We got up at the crack of dawn the next day and after tea in our room, caught an early train for London. We were lucky to get seats, and lucky in our companions. First was a blond Cockney girl who willingly answered all Dinah's questions with such a lovely accent. Then an elderly couple got on, typical upper-middle-class British, and they too were much taken with Dinah and practically adopted her. It was so like a story and everything so typical that I half expected to have to turn the page to see what was going to happen next.

The country was pretty and green, and wet of course. I was so glad that I got to England for autumn because at least the leaves here turn a little, and the countryside looks a little like fall.

The first night was pretty grim as no reservations had

been made for us and we had to find our own billets, but the next day we were taken to the billeting office, which is why I am at the Mount Royal. The hotel has a rather shady reputation but the lobby is fascinating with its variety of nationalities and polyglot conversations. And, one night as I was sitting there during an alert, reading a detective story, all of a sudden I realized that I was actually living in the town where the story took place, and that if I should get up and walk a few blocks, I could walk along the streets mentioned. It was a strange feeling—for so many years all my favorite books have been about England and many of them taken place in London and I have imagined myself there so often that it took time for me to realize that I was really there, not just in fancy.

I have written you about seeing Richard twice, I hope to see him this week again. He is most envious of me, and wishes that he too were departing. I don't think he is looking forward to another rainy cold winter here.

Your long letter, Father, of September 24th reached me here today. Thanks for the paternal advice, and I mean that sincerely. Even if I had liked Spain, I would probably had to have left as the embassy was cutting down on personnel. You, however, misinterpret my desire for discomfort. So far nothing that I have experienced has really been discomfort, merely more challenging living conditions. I dislike discomfort as much as anyone, but I enjoy comfort more when I have contributed to bringing it about. Does that make any sense? Remember the pillow I made for myself in North Africa? It would have been discomfort to have gone without a pillow entirely, but I appreciated a pillow a lot more because I made it myself; appreciated it a lot more than the one that came with my apartment in Madrid or even the one that I later bought. See what I mean?

Another thing is that I really enjoy having the Army around. I like the informality and friendliness that goes with it, something that one doesn't find in the other type of life.

Enough of that. Have I told you that one of my duties is to provide tea in the afternoon for the rest of the office? I must admit that I suggested it, but now that the habit has been added to our routine, I have no chance to back out and about four o'clock they begin to get restless. I think it is a wonderful custom and approve wholeheartedly.

After ten days of believing the sign saying that my kitchenette didn't work, I asked if it could be turned on, and found that it was on all the time. So yesterday I bought a cup and saucer, a plate, a saucepan and knife, fork and spoon. And today after a hasty lunch, I braved the complexities of coupons and went shopping for tonight's supper. Beside me as I type I have a burlap bag with little potatoes, Brussels sprouts, lettuce, bacon, mayonnaise and tomato soup powder, and a little apple. I already have a loaf of Hovis bread, orange marmalade, half a pint of milk, butter and cheese. So you can see that neither England nor I are exactly starving. I am looking forward immensely to my own home-cooked supper, something that I could never do in Spain as both Saturia and I would have lost face. I also have a John Buchan omnibus which I have not seen before and a new Dornford Yates which (maybe both) will be going to you, Father, as a Christmas present—after Richard has read them. . . .

Much, much love to all of you,

21 October 1944

Richard just wandered into the office with half a letter to me from you. By this time some of my letters should have gotten to you so you should know a little more about my plans—which is more than I do at the moment! The embassy is waiting final directions from Washington and then I will be on my way again. As I have said before, I am both sorry and glad, for I am enjoying my stay in London very much, but purely from a personal standpoint—there is not much work to do here and everything seems in a state of flux and change.

This letter is being written by a disillusioned person. For

years I have dreamed of having kippered herring for breakfast. I did this morning and I think the taste will be with me so long that dreaming will be unnecessary. What a bitter disappointment; I cannot see why so many of my favorite heroes like it so much.

Having lived in my apartment for so long without discovering that the electricity was on in the kitchenette, I am making up for lost time and having most of my suppers *chez moi*. It is such fun and I have found that it takes me less time to prepare and eat supper in my room than it does to wait until the dining room opens at seven, wait for the slow service and eat downstairs. And the dining room is such a dismal place to eat alone in. Even if one takes a book. And one always eats too many potatoes and the sweet for dessert is always hot, which continually surprises me.

I have not told you about my peregrinations of last Sunday . . . I started out up Oxford Street to Regent, down Regent window-shopping like mad in the windows of Liberty's and Jaeger's, across Pall Mall to the Mall, up the Strand until I got to St. Mary-le-Strand, a little church built on an island right in the middle of the street. It was eleven o'clock by then and the bells were ringing for the service, so I went in, and was very glad that I did, for it is a charming little church. After the service I walked on past the Law Courts, down Fleet Street and Ludgate Hill to St. Paul's. I was much disappointed in St. Paul's and went through it as a duty not as a pleasure. It is a big, cold empty place with no feeling of life or warmth to it. [As I realized years later this is true of most large churches; they come to life when one attends services.] Perhaps if I had taken my time and read all the inscriptions I would have felt differently, as it was I just made the circuit and came out. Then I found my way down to the river and walked up along the Embankment to Westminster Bridge, looked long at the Houses of Parliament and wished that it were spring and I knew someone so that I might have tea on the terrace, then up Birdcage Walk along

185

St. James Park to Buckingham Palace, with a quick side trip down to a sandwich bar by Victoria Station for a cup of tea and couple of sandwiches, and another brief stop in St. James Park to feed the crusts of my sandwiches to the ducks, swans and pigeons—and sparrows. I even got one sparrow to take a crumb right out of my hand. I was a bit footsore by that time and weary, so I came up through Green Park to Piccadilly, through Berkeley Square and back to Oxford Street. I then made the mistake of going to the movies, thinking that a spy picture called "Storm Over Lisbon" would be amusing, but it was awful and except for the first picture of the Commercial Square in Lisbon, it was not worth seeing. And so back to the hotel and supper, a book and early bed. Quite a Sunday. And, believe it or not, it didn't rain at all, not all day!

I'm surprised as I reread that letter that I made no mention of bomb damage. Was it that much of it came later from the V-2s, which were quite terrifying and just beginning? Was it that I didn't want to distress my family? Or was I perhaps wearing the rose-colored glasses of an Anglophile who had "come home," as it were?

28 October 1944

Dear Mother and Father:

My weekend with the Armstrongs [Jessie Aiken Armstrong and her second husband] was perfect. I knew it would be fun but I had no idea how simply wonderful. You know, it was the first time I had been in a house since I left the Andrés [in Algiers]. Only apartments and hotels in the intervening months. And it was the first time I had been really in the country [at night] since my tent days in Constantine and even that was noisy because of the convoys going by on the road all night. My room was up under the eaves and was lovely and cold, except for the bed which had a stone hot-water bottle in it to warm it up, and the night was so quiet that the silence was almost a positive thing, rather than just the absence of sound. Just the way moonlight shining on a floor is more intense when it is shining through a window so that the shadow of the window frame contrasts darkly with the brightness, so the silence was deeper because from time to time a leaf made a dry rustle as it was blown across the roof. And that, after the noises of the household had ceased, was the only sound I heard until the birds waked me in the morning. It was the first time since I was last in Chocorua that I had slept in such peaceful surroundings. No need to tell you how I loved it.

Perhaps I should go back and take the weekend in order. I had permission to leave the office a little early Saturday afternoon in order to catch a train shortly before four. But I got delayed at the last minute and waited fifteen minutes for a bus, finally took a taxi and made the train by a scant 30 seconds. I showed myself an inexperienced traveler by purchasing first-class tickets and of course had to stand in a third-class corridor. Apparently one buys third-class tickets, makes for first class carriages, and if a ticket conductor comes, which almost never happens, one pays the difference. Next time I will know better, but I really did not mind as standing I got a better view out the window than I would have sitting in a compartment.

A realization of the ever-presentness of the war here was brought home to me most strongly as I saw the gaping cellar holes, the little mounds in every backyard showing where the shelter was. Apparently neighbors vie with each other as to who has the prettiest shelter, for some of them are terraced and have flowers planted on top of them. But I couldn't seem to project myself in my imagination into the lives of people who have a bomb shelter just as they have a garage or a bathroom, and who have accepted a nightly migration into it as routinely as they used to put out the cat. It is incredible to me that they can seem as little touched by the war in that their sense of humor seems as keen as ever, their friendliness as warm as ever, and yet night after weary night they have lived like moles and the air and very earth around them has shaken with injury, death and destruction. I expected to find a nation of people with dull eyes and white hair (not literally of course) but life in London goes on much the same and even I have acquired a *blasé* attitude to the alerts. I was a little jumpy when I first came, and used to go down to the lobby to read instead of staying in my room, but now I am annoyed when they flash the signal on the movie screen as for a moment it interferes with the picture, and they don't even wake me at night. As far as I know I have heard nothing but the siren so far, but it is hard to be sure. And even the sirens are little used these days, which is a blessing as the blood-curdling wail of the sirens is a truly terrifying sound.

The war is still evident of course in the queues for everything, in the preponderance of women at such jobs as conductors on the trams and announcers at the stations and even porters at the stations. The latter impressed me immensely as generally they are not young at all and their ample figures have been stuffed into some sort of overalls and coats or jackets over that, and they are bustling around in the most cheery and helpful fashion, looking cold and wet part of the time but not so much so that they cannot crack a joke or two. But on the whole I have found austerity a good deal more pleasant than I had anticipated. (I really should not discuss the matter at all—reminds me of people who have been in China or someplace on a round-the-world tour and then dominate dinner conversations for years later with their views on China "when I lived there." So don't quote me, these are just my impressions and reactions during my brief, too brief, stay here.)

To get back to my weekend, I hung out the window at every stop to make sure that I didn't go past the one I wanted; I had to change twice and had no idea of the distance and the stations are poorly marked, so it was a bit nerve-wracking. Three Bridges was the first change, Pulborough the second and then a little shuttle to the station of Fittleworth, where the "taxi" met me. It was a short drive down narrow lanes in the twilight. The sun had been out for part of the day and as usual for part of the day it had rained, but now at sunset the sun was nearly through the clouds and gave a funny red glow to the fog and mist. And the air was incredibly soft and sweet-smelling, the hedges along the road were high and glistened with rain drops and the trees almost met over our heads. Sutton is a tiny little village with a pub on the corner of two roads and a mere handful of houses and the church. Jessie (I call her Mrs. Armstrong to her face) has a cottage just out of the village, built up above the road so that one has to climb up steep steps to the higher land above and the quince tree in her garden hangs down over the road below. I never would have recognized her, but we felt congenial at once and after she had shown me to my room and I had washed up a bit, I met Mr. Armstrong and the three of us walked down the road to a friend's house where we had been invited for a drink before dinner. I, of course, joined into the conversation very little but sat content in front of an open fire (months and months since I had seen one) and listened to them talk, thinking that it was just like one of Angela Thirkell's books and that one of the delightful things was that everyone was so in character and said just what one expected them to. There was the Scots doctor who had spent years in East Africa, and his maiden sister who had just been miraculously cured of her liver trouble by a woman who comes to the village and who sounds like a combination of an osteopath and a Christian Scientist. And there were the host and hostess who are well enough off and come "to the country" for weekends to drink and play golf, yet who are really much nicer than that description would make them sound.

Dinner cooking at home took us back after about an hour and the three of us walked arm in arm with only the starlight and a sliver of a new moon to light us home. Dinner was good and afterwards (no dishwashing at night) we sat in front of the fire with their beautiful Persian cat on the hearth at our feet, and talked and I showed them pictures of the family and those lovely ones of Italy that you sent me the other day (and which I shall use as Christmas cards. I was amazed, I didn't know that I took such good pictures!) About ten-thirty we all of us yawned and decided it was bedtime and I retired to my pleasant night's sleep.

Breakfast was a late and leisurely affair and then I had the fun of helping with the dishes and the beds, and found that two years away from those domestic chores had in no way impaired the rapid flow of conversation which I used to help pass the time. And Mrs. Armstrong had apparently been lost without young David in the house. He is away at boarding school, and so she was most eager for company and someone to talk to as well as listen to. And I do think I did almost my share of listening. We both went into the village with my ration book and I gave the shopkeeper my month's sweets ration for Jessie's use, no hardship to me and apparently pleased Jessie very much and impressed the shopkeeper no end. I also took some PX candy for David, some cigarettes for Mr. Armstrong and stuff like cold cream, talcum powder, soap and tea for Jessie and Joan. Little things but apparently appreciated and welcome. We also called on the Scots doctor, then Jessie had to get back to a custard that was baking and I went for a walk through a muddy lane, across a field and down by a noisy little brook, across the bridge and up a hill to the next village. I stood for minutes on end on the bridge listening to the chatter of the water over the stones, listening to crows in the next field and even conversing for a moment with a gray squirrel that stopped to pass the time of day with me. There were still flowers blooming (sent under separate cover a few days ago), the sun was out most of the time, chickadees kept me company part of the way through a little wood and best of all, when I got to the top of the hill and saw the village, I discovered that they actually do have thatched houses in England and that it wasn't all a myth invented by the *National Geographic* and the postcard people. It was really quite exciting and I stood and looked at the house I liked best so long that I was afraid the boy sawing wood down the road would get suspicious and think I was a German spy or something. I also saw a typical English squire in plus-fours and argyle socks with heavy shoes, carrying a stick and accompanied by a lovely setter. I took a couple of pictures and got very muddy and hot and hungry before I got back just in time for dinner. Which also was a good meal, with a roast and even two kinds of dessert!

We did the dishes again and sat in front of the fire knitting for a little while, then Jessie and I went for a walk, leaving Mr. A. taking a nap. I forgot to tell you that the whole house was filled with the heavenly fragrance of the apples and quince that they had picked the day before. I brought a quince back to town with me and my room too has a little of the same sharp, clean smell.

Just think of it, I spent Sunday afternoon walking on the downs. Magic word, I had read it so many times and imagined doing just that, yet never thought that I would. They weren't quite as I had thought they were, less grass and more wooded areas, but still pretty wonderful. We walked up a lane called Puck's Street, the lower half of which was almost a brook (later we discovered that David and Mr. Armstrong had once built a dam and diverted the brook from its channel across the road, and ever since the brook had shown a tendency to wander). Higher up the woods were mostly beech trees, and, with both the ground covered with the yellow leaves and the trees still thickly hung with them, it was like walking in a golden glow. The leaves underfoot were too wet to scuffle the way leaves should in the fall, but it was generally pretty satisfactory and it felt good to walk on them and it smelt good to be among them. There is little red in an English autumn, but there were just enough mountain ash and sumac to give a crimson contrast to the yellows and browns. And the view on top was superb. We talked a blue streak all the time, though I cannot remember just what about. Coming home we met three kittens who bounced out of their barnyard to be petted and then followed us crying for almost a mile.

A young man, rare person in England these days, had been asked in for tea. I picked some lovely smoky blue asters (they call them Michaelmas daisies here), put an apple in my pocket, packed my bag and left on the 6:15 train, very reluctantly I must admit. The trouble with the whole weekend was that it was too nice and made me so homesick for Chocorua. Jessie is a darling, her husband most pleasant and both of them extremely hospitable. I am sorry that I shan't be able to see them again before I go. Jessie has taken up pencil drawing and has done some really lovely little things. I persuaded her that you would love one as a Christmas card.

Oh, I forgot to tell you that en route to the train a perfect V of geese, seven or nine of them there were, flew very low over the car. I had never seen geese flying so low before and it was an impressive sight.

The train ride back was pleasant, but the Underground [subway] quite an experience. Me in it for the first time alone and with my arms loaded with my suitcase, *New Yorker,* umbrella and a big bunch of flowers.

Enough of this for this time. Must stop.

Elizabeth

31 October 1944

Dear Mother and Father:

Richard and I had a most delightful weekend in the country together, and I got him to take me to see the duck pond that he used to write about. That was Sunday afternoon and after lunch we got a couple of bicycles and rode over. Fortunately, it didn't rain at all and the sun even came out from time to time. But it was pretty cold and we were glad of the exercise to keep warm. And Sunday night we went to the pub that is practically a second home for the boys, pleasant but not remarkable. The weekend was really a quiet one, and sitting in the officers' lounge reading was what we did most of the time. As Christopher Robin said to Pooh, what he really liked to do best was nothing. Pooh wanted to know what doing nothing was and Christopher Robin said it was when someone asked you what you were going to do and you said, oh nothing, and then you went and did it. That is the kind of weekend it was most of the time. It was fun seeing so much of Richard.

Excuse the briefness but time is short and my activities many. Among other things I am going to Berlitz two hours a day! Quite strenuous.

8 November 1944

Dear Mother and Father:

Give my love to our tall friend [my boss in Madrid] when you see him. I miss him.

Discouraging business, this waiting for visas and travel orders and things. Here I still am—and everyone expected I would have been away two weeks ago. But now I should be hardened to this sort of thing, the "what, are you still here" attitude of one's friends and colleagues. But the exhausting part is trying to have clean clothes ready at all times. One by one I have got my shirts and blouses all washed and ironed, and now I don't dare wear them. The climax will come at the end of this week when I wash and iron the last pair of pajamas, and will then have to sleep with nothing on as I am saving a clean pair to wear on my voyages. Part of the hardships of war, don't you know.

Joan Aiken [Jessie Aiken Armstrong's daughter] and I got together finally and I had dinner with her and her fiancé Ron. We had a heavenly meal with roast beef even, and then sat around the fireplace with the kitten and talked and toasted our toes. She is a darling, smaller even than Jane and with the same lovely hair. Ron is a peach of a fellow and seems devoted to her.

Sunday I slept late, made my own breakfast of tea and toast with orange marmalade and then went out to Hampstead by the tube to walk around the town and over the Heath. I didn't remember it very well, but one particular spot where I seem to recollect very clearly watching sheep grazing, I found covered with *objets de la guerre*. Most depressing. The day was gray and windy and later blew up to squalls of rain, but I had over an hour with only occasional spatters of rain and came back to London feeling very rosy-cheeked and healthy. Richard called just after I got back and asked me to come over to his new flat; you knew that he had moved to town, didn't you? He lured me with the prospect of an open fire and an iron, so I put all the odds and ends of groceries I had in the kitchen into my shopping bag, and put all my washed, still wet and unironed laundry into my suitcase, and braved the elements from the interior of a cab. Liz, his (or should I say one of his) English girls, was there darning his socks when I arrived, so I set myself up in the kitchen and ironed for over an hour. Liz had to leave early, so the three of us had tea by the fire and then I cooked supper for Richard and myself - cabbage with butter and cream (milk to you), boiled potatoes, little sausages, and a tomato, celery and lettuce salad with a piece of cheese for dessert. Very satisfactory and Richard was properly appreciative. He has a most attractive flat in a mews [what were formerly stables in a small street or alley now converted into apartments], a big living room and kitchen on the ground floor with big windows looking out into the alley, and upstairs two bedrooms and a bath. Reminded me very much of Rollins Place [on Beacon Hill in Boston where I had lived before going overseas]; the atmosphere was much the same.

No other news worth writing about. I wish you two would realize that even letters sent to the wrong or no-longer-correct address will be forwarded to me. I cannot understand this chit-chat about waiting for a permanent address before you write!

194

The mail situation was really getting me down; on October 31, I wrote about receiving letters from them mailed in September, so it was no wonder I was a bit repetitious in my requests. Yet one dated November 9, 1944 and addressed to me "Care of Mail Room Department of State" arrived days later, so obviously someone knew where to reach me. Signed for the Secretary of State by G. Howland Shaw, an assistant secretary, it was stamped SECRET in large red letters, and read as follows:

My dear Miss Phenix: The Department of State informs you that you have been designated as Clerk at the American Legation at Bern, Switzerland. Separate instructions concerning your assignment have been issued to the Legation at Bern.

And so I was off again. This time I was allowed only 65 pounds of baggage and so had to do an enormous amount of repacking and readdressing all the boxes my mother had been sending me in preparation of a long, cold winter in London with severe rationing of clothing and other necessities.

I arrived in Paris on November 13 and days later wrote home in part:

Dear Mother and Father:

The [plane] trip over was uneventful: seeing the cold green water beneath me made me think of the usual six seasick hours that one had to endure [on the Channel ferry]. I "picked up" a middle-aged technical expert on the trip into the city, as he said he was looking for the embassy and I offered to guide him—result, a date with him that night. We wandered around in the gentle rain for over an hour and won the eternal love of a *gendarme* of whom I asked directions [in French, of course]. He said we were a quarter of an hour away from the Rond Point and I replied what did it matter, it was Paris! Whereupon, I thought he would kiss me on both cheeks, but he didn't. We ended up in a nightclub, saw a good floor show, drank better than fair champagne. My escort got a bit tight, and when he said goodnight to me at the door of the Hotel Gallia, he said he had had a good time but was a bit disappointed because he had planned to spend $200 and had only spent $30!

I have many friends here and have been leading a gay life. Keeler Faus is up from Madrid, Harry Woodruff is here, Mr. Chapin's [the ambassador's] secretary was a friend of mine in Algiers, and then there are many others. We had a small Algiers party last night and went to a restaurant for couscous, that wonderful Algerian dish. And another night I met a nice Pfc [Private First Class] and we spent the evening in a bar (the three places in Paris where you don't get too cold are bars, cinemas and the Métro), drinking Martinis. And another night Keeler took me to the movies. Oh, I forgot to tell you that our 'mess' [where we eat] is at the Crillon! It really is the most curious combination here of luxury and hardship. Rather amusing, sometimes, the women in fur coats and elaborate hats and coiffures, riding bicycles. The bicycle cabs in which many women do their shopping. The horse cabs and the pony carts. The windows filled with every sort of merchandise, perfumes, silks, fur coats, crazy hats— and all crazy prices. The assortment of clothes that most people wear to keep warm. And above all, the feeling of remoteness from the war—no real blackout, no air raids, no sudden noises in the night; only the uniforms to remind you, only the bullet-scarred buildings and the wreaths of flowers on corners of the Place de la Concorde, in memory of those who died there that Paris might be free. It is a most unreal city and soap-bubble place, and for that reason the discomforts are accepted with less grace than they are in London or Algiers or any other place that seems closer to the war.

I've done a lot of sleeping, a fair amount of eating, a reasonable amount of drinking, and a terrific amount of walking. I've been much interested at how much my memory brought back to me. Wednesday, I found my way with no trouble at all to Aunt Rose's apartment on the Rue de Varenne. [She was the widow of Robert E. Olds, formerly an undersecretary of state with whom my father had worked when we lived in Washington. I spent the summer of my freshman year in college with her in Paris—very carefully chaperoned.] Tell her the street looks the same as ever and they still sell cabbages in the greengrocers on the Rue de Bac. Then I walked up to St. Germain de Prés (past Les Deux Magots, [the well-known cafe], of course) and down the river again where I watched the men fishing from the banks and where I lingered among the bookstalls.

Yesterday I walked down the Rue de Rivoli, pushing my way through piled-up vegetables on the sidewalk (beets, carrots, cabbages, celery, turnips, lettuce and even artichokes), down to the Île de la Cité. Notre Dame is still, in my mind, the loveliest cathedral I've seen, and by this time I've seen a number. My favorite pottery store is still there and I bought a Quimper ashtray as my souvenir of Paris. And a number of really lovely postcards. Tomorrow, if the weather clears a little, I shall go to Montmartre. And Sunday I leave bright and early, (well, early anyway) with the courier. A long and very cold trip I expect.

My family heard from me next via an RCA Radiogram dated November 22, 1944: "Arrived after pleasant trip address American Legation Berne how about some mail love Elizabeth Phenix."

CHAPTER SEVEN

The End of an Era

❖

November 22, 1944–August 5, 1945

Through the autumn, Allied armies continued to advance across Europe, until mid-December when German counterattacks in the Ardennes Forest of Belgium marked the beginning of the Battle of the Bulge. The U.S. Army broke the siege of Bastogne on December 26, the German counteroffensive failed and the defeat of the Third Reich appeared inevitable, thus ending Hitler's threat of an empire that would last a thousand years.

In February 1945, Berlin was bombed by 1,000 U.S. planes, and British Lancasters firebombed Dresden with phosphorus and high-explosive ordinance, killing an estimated 135,000 inhabitants.

On April 12, while vacationing at Warm Springs, President Franklin D. Roosevelt suffered a cerebral hemorrhage and died. Vice President Harry Truman was sworn in as president.

Germany surrendered to the Allies at Rheims in France on May 7, and May 8 was officially declared V-E Day.

In the Pacific on July 30 a Japanese submarine sank the *U.S.S. Indianapolis*, which had just completed a top-secret mission to deliver to the island of Tinian the cores of two atomic bombs destined to be dropped on Japan.

Although I could have done with a day or two of settling in professionally and personally, it was very good to be needed and to be put to work at once as one of the secretaries in Allen Dulles's office. But it was a week before I was able to supplement my cable with a proper letter, bringing my parents up to date with my activities in Paris and recounting the adventures of my trip to Bern with the courier.

29 November 1944

Dear Mother and Father:

My last letter to you was ten days ago, written in an office that my Pfc. friend borrowed for me. (His name is Patrick Fitzpatrick, for your information, and one of the brightest people I have met in a long time. Made my stay in Paris so much nicer, having someone so congenial to play around with.) Saturday was a lovely warm sunny day, the first one we had had since I had gotten there, and I sat on a bench in the sun under the sycamore trees along the Champs Elysées for almost half an hour. Saturday afternoon I moved down to the Crillon, as I was leaving early the next morning and the Gallia was too far away, with all my bags. The Crillon is still very luxurious and my room had a tremendous private bathroom, up three steps from the bedroom. Saturday night in Paris is really bath night, as we have hot water then (and theoretically all day Sunday too but not always) and many of the Americans turn down parties and such to go home and take a bath. I paid back a little of the debt I owed from my North African days, when my favorite dates were those with bathtubs and hot water, and told Pat to bring a towel over when he came to get me after supper, so that he could take a bath! Being an enlisted man, he gets even less hot water. Also being an enlisted man, we could never eat together, which several times resulted in our not eating at all! I was too sleepy and too journey-proud to be very gay that night, so we merely had a few drinks in the Crillon bar and then I sent him home. It is a nuisance the way one seems to meet the nicest people under shipboard circumstances.

Breakfast in solitary splendor in the big Crillon dining

room the next morning at 7:30 and then I met the courier across the street at the Embassy. We left promptly at eight and for a wonder the weather was again pleasant. Two days in a row in Paris in November is unbelievable. Our transportation was the Army vehicle known as a command car and there were the driver, the State Department courier, the guard and myself. It was a long drive across France, but of course most interesting—my only wish was that we had been in a Jeep so that I could have seen out better. But that would have been too cold. The back seat of a command car is not the smoothest riding in the world, but is not too bad. We stopped outside of a town about halfway there for lunch in a sort of station restaurant—apparently they always stop there and are expected on certain days. Sometime I shall have to amuse you with the tale of me looking for the W.C. and of what I found out back of the chicken yard.

I did remember to tell them: I had asked in my best correct French *"Où est le lavabo, s'il vous plaît?"* The response was to show me a small washbasin in the hall between the dining room and the kitchen. So I tried again *"Non merci, où est le W.C.?"* i.e. "water closet," what one calls a toilet in France. And I was shown out the back door, through the vegetable garden, past the chickens to a small shack with a hole in the ground and two concrete footprints on which to stand. A closet of sorts but certainly not a water closet! I wished I had known my masculine traveling companions well enough to have shared the episode with them.

I went on to write:

We drove through Fontainebleau and I could catch a glimpse of the chateau through the trees. I thought back to the time that I was there with Aunt Rose. I had hoped that we would go through Dijon but we went a little north of it. About three o'clock we could see mountains with snow on them far off on the horizon, and about dusk we reached them. Pontarlier had about a foot of snow and I could only wish that it was daylight so that I could see more of the surroundings than our headlights lit up. It was rather exciting, crossing the frontier at night, getting out of the car into the deep snow and stumbling across to the guard house to show our passports, then the gates were raised and we drove into no-man's-land right up to the Swiss gates. There I expected a little difficulty, because my visa was for entry by way of Geneva as I had not expected to come with the courier, but I had practiced what I was going to say in French all day and the assurances that the Swiss consulate in Paris had given me permission (which they had, on the phone) rolled smoothly off my tongue and the guard, instead of questioning my entry, welcomed me to Switzerland with a charming smile and a warmly hospitable greeting.

Another car was waiting for us the other side of the Swiss gates, and we offloaded the pouches and said goodbye to our military driver and guard. The still cold night, the stars, the feel and smell of the snow and the crunch of it under my feet made me both homesick for Chocorua (it has been almost three years since I have seen any amount of snow) and at the same time exhilarated me. My emotions about coming here have been mixed, while as you know I don't like being stationed in a neutral country during wartime, still I have always wanted to go to Switzerland and I couldn't help being excited about that.

We drove to the station and checked some of the bags and pouches and then went to the station hotel restaurant for supper while we waited for our train. The taxi-driver bought me a glass of vermouth, the chef came out to shake hands with me and welcome me to Switzerland, the people in the restaurant all smiled at me, and right from the beginning I felt that this was a much more *simpático* country than Spain. And to make everything quite wonderful, we had venison for supper, the first time that I have ever had it. I didn't recognize the word in French and the taxi driver explained it by telling me about the forests and the hunting that one could do here.

The train ride was anticlimactic; one could see nothing of the country through which we passed and both the courier and I were quite tired. But it was strange to catch glimpses of snow-covered stations and to hear the soft Swiss-German that is spoken in this part of the country. It took a little adjustment for me to remember that I didn't have to glare at a person, just because he spoke German!

We got into Bern about eleven o'clock, a car from the legation met us, and I told them to choose just any hotel that had beds and hot water. They dropped me off at the Bellevue on their way up to the legation, and again I was impressed by the hospitality of the people. A pleasant desk clerk personally escorted me to my room, a pink-cheeked chambermaid came right in to open my bed and ask if there was anything she could do for me. (I assured her that all I wanted was to sleep and she couldn't do that for me—even the bath didn't seem important, which was lucky, as the hot water goes off shortly after nine.)

Monday was clear and sunny and from where I sat in the dining room for breakfast I could see the snowy mountains beyond the city. I was lucky to have had that one sunny day to welcome me, for the rest of the week was rainy and gray.

They don't waste any time here, and I was at work Monday afternoon! There are two other girls in the office with me, both of them just as nice as they can be, and we are most congenial. One of them is the sister of a boy I knew in Algiers! She is getting married in the near future and I am planning to take over her apartment in the old part of town. It has inconveniences, like no bathtub, but the personality of the place and its charm make up for the inconveniences I think, and will make it more fun living there than in the modern impersonal flat I looked at yesterday in the district up beyond the legation. After all, most of the time that I have been overseas I have done very well without a bathtub,

203

and with less compensation. I'll write you all about it when and if I move into it. I am at present still living in the Belle-vue, which is rather expensive but most agreeable. The manager sent me a dish of fruit night before last, to soften the blow of the bill which I got the next morning, I think! I eat breakfast every morning in the big dining room with its view across the river to the hills and mountains (when you can see them) and the waiter and I are old friends by now. I so much prefer the Continental breakfast of *café au lait* (no sugar, very strictly rationed here) and a roll with sweet butter and maybe a bit of honey or marmalade.

Lunch I make my big meal and eat at one of the many restaurants. One has to pay two meal coupons for every meal, sometimes three if the meal is very large or uses a lot of rationed food. Rationing here is much more complicated than in London, but one has the feeling that it is a preventative measure rather than an actual necessity. Clothing is rationed and shoes, of course, but so are milk and cheese and chocolate, things that I had expected to find plentiful.

Supper I am now having *chez moi*. Fortunately I was smart enough to bring my little Sterno stove with me, so I bought a little saucepan and made bouillon with the cubes I brought from England. Then I sometimes save a piece of rye bread from lunch, and yesterday I learned I could buy a sort of rye crisp with some meal coupons, so last night I feasted with some cheese that one of the girls had given me coupons for, rye crisp, bouillon and one of the manager's apples. Work begins late here, we have a long lunch hour and so we work rather late in the evenings. Between having had a large lunch and being tired by the time I get through in the evening, dinner in the dining room with a lot of people does not appeal to me and I get along much better with a light supper in my room, and an hour of reading. I brought almost twenty pounds of books with me—right now I am reading the Helen McInnes, which is quite good but nowhere near up to her others.

I daren't write any more. Just add that the things I need here most are as already requested: multivitamin pills, underwear panties with elastic tops, some more soap (Ivory) and perhaps sugar lumps! And canned butter, one of the girls has suggested.

5 December 1944

Dear Mother and Father:

Bern is such a charming little city. You can walk from one end to the other in no time at all, yet it is so full of so many unexpected corners and side streets that it will take some time to know every bit of it. A week ago Sunday I went on an exploring walk which lasted more than two hours. Have you got a map so that you can see the general layout of the town? The old part is on a rocky peninsula around which the river Aare rushes. My hotel is almost on the edge on one side and I have to cross a high bridge over the river every morning. It is fun to watch the different colors and moods of the water that runs so swiftly underneath. It always looks very cold and very swift, but sometimes it is green and sometimes blue and sometimes sort of muddy if it has been raining much. Sunday I crossed the bridge as if I were going to the office but then turned upstream for a quarter of a mile and walked back right on the edge of the river under the bridge and down to the bridge that crosses from the end of the peninsula. The town stands on the very edge of the water, so close to the water that when the river was very full two weeks ago it flowed over its banks and some of the lowest houses had to be evacuated.

I crossed back into town and walked up the hill under the arcade. In this old part of the city all the streets are arcades and one can keep dry in the worst weather. It makes window shopping more difficult, however, because the shops have displays on both sides of the sidewalk and I get dizzy trying to see both at the same time.

The people are very friendly and helpful and very good at

205

understanding my French. All these languages are getting me confused and the Swiss-German that is spoken here doesn't help at all. My pet expression, and one that is used all the time here, is *Merci vielmals*! Did I tell you that I took German lessons at Berlitz when I was in London? Not many, just enough to start bringing back to mind the two years of German that I had in college. So I mix French and German, add a word of Italian and a couple of phrases in Spanish just to confuse people, and get along really very well. Asked at lunch the other day if I wanted anything to drink, I replied: *"Gracias, seulement wasser."* And I got it too!

Sunday afternoon four of us climbed the large hill or small mountain, depending on one's point of view, that is just beyond the town. There is supposedly quite good skiing on it in the deep of winter. And it makes a lovely walk with breathtaking views all the way up and from the top. The woods are still quite autumnly, the sun was out for the first time since I had come (rains as much as it does in London, I think) and the fields are still green, yet the mountains in the distance are capped with snow. Much as I am looking forward to the snow and the winter, I am already impatient for the spring, which must be incredibly lovely here. Already in my imagination I have filled every bowl in my not-yet-acquired apartment with plants and flowers and ferns and things picked in the woods that are within such easy walking distance of the town. It is so nice to be in a town that has shops and theatres and movies and restaurants and all the other things that one wants from a town, and yet be so close to the country that you don't even need to take a train to get there, you can walk or take a tram. Just the way I like to live best.

Some of the days are quite cold now, one morning as I walked to work there was a heavy white frost on the grass and trees and covering the barberry bushes by the river, so that they gleamed white and bright red. The town is getting ready for Christmas and the windows are full of presents and decorated with angels and Christmas trees and stars and tinsel. It has been a long time since I have seen so many nice things and have been in the middle of holiday preparations. That is one reason why I am so eager to find an apartment soon so that I can buy a wreath and perhaps even a Christmas tree. I have already bought some little figures for a crèche. Oh, and they have the most delicious marzipan and *lebekuchen* made like bears or other animals.

Now listen—I went skiing last weekend! Up to a place in the mountains called Kleine Scheidegg. Most of the day we skied in the clouds, but just before lunch they all blew away and for a moment we could see the Matterhorn in the distance. I had to pinch myself to make myself believe that I was really there.

I stayed on a little slope all day, just trying to get the feel of skis again, and got so I could do a pretty good *Christiana* to the right. I rented the skis at the hotel and they were very satisfactory. It is much more important to have good boots than to have good skis.

We lunched with friends at the hotel, had coffee in front of an open fire and then went out again. The day was made more amusing by the irrepressible Air Corps boys (they were of course internees) who were all over the slopes. Many of them had never skied before and they were loud and noisy and very American in their attempts to learn. I of course got to talking with them (my Red Cross background perhaps) and one of them commented on how well I spoke English, almost like an American! Then when they discovered that I really was an American, they nearly died of excitement. At lunch I could hear them pointing me out as the girl who had spoken to them and who was an *American girl,* and later on the slope again a nice redhead came up to me saying he had heard I was from Boston and that he was from Belmont! It was a lot of fun, a dozen or more of them crowded into the same car with us on the train on the way back, they wanted to know when we were coming skiing again, wanted us to promise to come to their Christmas dance, and practically talked our ears off. It is so easy to be popular with that age and group—all you have to do is to be a sympathetic listener and they think you are wonderful.

We had tea before we left at five o'clock, when it was getting dark, and got back to Bern about 8:30, in time to take advantage of the evening allowance of hot water, and to fall into bed. I found that I did much more skiing after I was in bed than I had done all day, my outraged muscles refusing to relax and let me sleep. But I was only a little stiff the next morning. And very pleased with my weekend.

13 December 1944

Dear Mother and Father:

You should see Bern this morning! It snowed softly all night long and when I got up this morning every tree and bush had turned white and as I walked down the street, at the far end the spire of the big church was misty gray against the lavender gray sky. And everything was very quiet and hushed—strange the way snow seems to absorb noises so that the world seems more silent.

I have finally moved into an apartment, only a temporary residence until I can move into Betty's. The hotel was much too expensive albeit very pleasant. My present domicile is just around the corner from the office and therefore extremely convenient.

Shopping for things to eat here is most amusing. First of all, it calls for so many French words that I don't know. For instance I know of course what bread is, but I didn't know what a loaf of bread was. And then everything is in liters and grams and kilos. I went in to buy a loaf of bread and was asked how many grams I wanted! They just don't teach the right things at school, I guess. And butter, I knew how big a piece but had no idea how many grams it would be. And of course, all the ration coupons are made out according to grams, so it is important that one figure things out on that scale. But most confusing. I have a nice blue string bag and come back after lunch every day looking very domestic with paper parcels sticking out the holes of the bag and maybe a bunch of carrots topping the whole thing off. It is lots of fun and I have to be very stern with myself that I don't buy things just for the sake and pleasure of buying. I had Mildred [another secretary in the office] to supper the first night I was in the apartment, and we feasted very well on a little already-cooked chicken that I bought and some BirdsEye peas. The BirdsEye place is right across the street, so I slip out of the office about 6:30 and buy what I need.

Coffee is so strictly rationed here that as far as I can see, it is impossible to have it for breakfast every day. And tea is the same. So I have found a little tea room where they serve a delicious *café complet* and I eat breakfast there every morning (except Mondays and Tuesdays, when they are closed). About three cups of *café au lait*, two or three slices of dark bread, reasonably adequate serving of butter and last week the most heavenly blueberry jam! All for about thirty cents. Two pleasant girls run the place and I am now greeted like an old and favored customer. There must be children in the family, back in the kitchen, for all during breakfast one morning I heard very young voices singing *"Sur le pont d'Avignon."* The girls are French but even so they mix their languages up and it still amuses me to hear them greet the milkman with a *Grüss Gott* and then add *Merci* as they take the milk!

I had loads of mail day before yesterday, Monday being mail day, and my morale was accordingly raised. And then there was a book from Richard that had been following me around for months and two *New Yorkers* (the subscription is expiring, will you renew it please), a *Cosmopolitan* and two Sunday Times (which I am saving for this Sunday.) Quite a haul, wasn't it, and I was the most popular girl in the office, with all that reading material. The Boss [Allen Dulles] has been quite low in spirits with an attack of gout, so I gave him one of the *New Yorkers* to cheer him up. It did, too.

It is quite different, this office from others I have worked in. In some ways more formal, in some ways less, but the thing that characterizes it most is that in spite of the fact that our hours are not nine to five, the attitude is a nine-to-five attitude, if you know what I mean. And a definite lack of enthusiasm. But I like the Boss and my two associates couldn't be nicer. And of course I love the country and the snow and the town and everything.

20 December 1944

Dear Mother and Father:

This last weekend was a gay one. Mildred and I went to the movies together Saturday night. Sunday morning I slept late and then had a luxurious breakfast of toast, butter and marmalade, lots of *café au lait*, a poached egg on toast and bacon! I got my supplementary rations (given when one moves from a hotel into an apartment) and among other items, I got six eggs! The usual monthly ration is one or two. So I am going to hardboil two of them and write Merry Christmas on them with colored pencil and give them as Christmas presents to two of the boys who are coming in for a drink *chez moi* before the reception Sunday night. And I read the October 1st Sunday Times. Then about noon I went for a long walk with my camera up and down the streets of the old section of town and even up the tower of the Protestant cathedral. It was a clear sunny day and the mountains were out for the first time in weeks. Unfortunately the horizon was too cloudy to make pictures of the mountains possible. Saturday night all the shops had stayed open later than usual and the windows were decorated with holly and balsam boughs. Did I tell you that all along the main street during the week there are vegetable and fruit and flower stalls and that one can do all one's marketing of that sort in the open air? Now Christmas trees and wreaths and holly and mistletoe have been added to their stocks and it is too gay for words. The big square by the bridge has a forest of little balsam trees all around the main fountain, many of the trees lightly dusted with snow, and the smell is heavenly. Children proudly drag their tree away and up the hill and at lunch time the other day a little boy, his cheeks pink with the cold and his school bag strapped across his shoulders, stood feeding the pigeons that swarmed around him and even lit on his shoulders. He was completely oblivious of the people passing by and surrounded as he was by the Christmas trees, he might have been completely alone in the woods. I wished that I had had my camera with me, that I might have taken his picture.

About two in the afternoon I realized that it was meal time again and went home to cook my lunch of tiny carrots, little boiled potatoes and canned tongue. And then I got ready for the tea dance given by the *Grande Société de Berne*, to which I had been invited. It was quite an affair, the society is over 200 years old and all that time has met in the same place. Everybody that is anybody was there, both Bernese and diplomatic, and I had a heavenly time. Everybody danced with me and I met many people and it was really much fun. I was taken by a member of the club, one of the Americans here, but even so I had to be passed on by the committee!

I was much interested to hear that Mary Elizabeth and her family are moving. [In Madrid, the ambassador was being transferred. His replacement was apparently less embarrassed by having "spooks" literally on his doorstep.]

27 December 1944

Dear Mother and Father:

Merry Christmas and Happy New Year and all that sort of thing. I'm afraid the cable I sent a couple of days ago was delayed—there was quite a holiday rush at the telegraph office. How did you like the one from the Boss? [It read "Merry Christmas to Evelyn and you. Your daughter well doing splendid work. Allen Dulles."] Pure guff, he dictated it to me and then asked me to work Sunday! And Monday too, so I didn't have much time to be homesick in. He said he thought you would like to know that I was taken care of over the holidays! Kind of him, what?

Pre-Christmas preparations were much the best part of Christmas this year. I was just as glad to be working, because it really did save me from being homesick. Both for the Christmas I had with you two years ago and the one I had last year, which was such fun. Remember how we decorated the tree with Necco wafers and Life Savers? And how Doug and two Italian soldiers practically tore down a pine tree along the highway that I might have evergreen boughs to make a wreath for our front door? Sometimes I regret very much my decision to leave the Red Cross, but I really had no choice, circumstances being what they were.

I bought a very pretty little tree this year and some holly, and had planned to spend all Sunday fixing up the apartment, heating the front room and so forth. And then I had to work, which made things a little hectic that evening, as I was having people in for cocktails before going to the reception given at the minister's house. My guests had to work as late as I did, so I made them help me when I got home. I had found figures for a crèche nowhere near as pretty as the ones I got in Italy last year, but not bad from a distance. And the two boys I had invited brought silver balls and bells to put on the tree, and I had icicles, so it really looked very gay when we were through with it. Red candles in the window and holly in the table and even a few presents under the tree. The Boss brought us each a bottle of perfume from Paris, Mildred gave me a charming pottery pitcher, Betty gave me some little linen cocktail napkins, and one of the other girls gave me a pretty box of cookies. So for a gal just recently come here, I had a nice pile of packages under my tree.

Five or six of us went to midnight Mass at the Catholic Church after the party, something I have long wanted to do, but it was very disappointing. Extremely crowded and cold and long. But the walk home was beautiful, a clear cold night with many stars, the steeple of the cathedral all lit up and, to make it all the more unreal, we could even hear the dull distant sounds of guns. Incredible but true, because of the combination of night and cold and wind.

I worked all day Monday too and Monday night the Boss had a buffet supper at his house, a very pleasant and successful one. A lovely Christmas tree, with candles and sparklers right on the tree, on the table and delicious food. Consommé, salad and rolls and cold meat and chicken and goose and olives and pickles, then canned apricots and the most wonderful chocolate cake with chocolate caramel roses and whipped cream and nuts and frosting on top. Then champagne in the living room and some of the boys played the piano and we sang songs for almost two hours. Then one of them (named Deforest Spencer, his father used to be commercial attaché in Vienna in the early 1930s, did you ever know him?) played classical pieces, many of those that you play, Father, and he did them almost as well, and I got so homesick I almost wept. He is an awfully pleasant chap. Had three years at Harvard and lived in Leverett House, knows Dr. [Leigh] Hoadley [master of Leverett House and a summer neighbor in Chocorua] of course. His family comes from St. Paul but I am sure that we must be distant cousins of some sort.

So you can see that it was a gay weekend, and can understand why it is a little difficult to concentrate on the job today. Both Betty and Mildred were away (it is my turn next weekend, and I have been solemnly informed by the Boss that broken legs are forbidden for the duration) so I had the fun of the office and the Boss to myself. Very nice, and gregarious as I am, I really prefer it that way. One gets more work done more quickly and there is much more the feeling of working with rather than for him.

I should have lots to write about next week—did I tell you where I was going? Three whole days at Davos, which is up near St. Moritz and supposed to be just wonderful. I can hardly wait for the week to end.

2 January 1945

Dear Mother and Father:

Those previous indications of filial devotion are as nothing compared to this one (I have at hand Father's comments on the subject). Here it is seven o'clock and for once the Boss has gone off at a reasonable hour and everyone else has left. Yet I stay on, to write my weekly epistle home. Aren't you impressed? You see, what you don't seem to understand is that letters can never, or almost never, be written during the working day, so one must either get here early or stay late. And the reason I usually wait until Wednesday morning is so that the news can be as up to the minute as possible; if I wrote the letter Saturday or even Monday, all the things that happened up to Wednesday [the day personal mail was sent out by diplomatic pouch] would have to remain until the next week, by which time they might be crowded out of my mind by more recent things. So there, for your remarks about procrastination and such. It is not any such thing, just thoughtfulness and intelligent planning. Of course. What else could you expect from me?

Also a big package of books from Richard—from you I mean via Richard. Many thanks; it is a wealthy feeling to have a shelf full of unread books. Much more satisfying than money in the bank. And also my Christmas packages. The little diary goes into my pocketbook and the big New England one lies open on my desk for all to admire, and to make me homesick. The balsam pillow will go to bed with me, to give me sweet dreams. I love the material.

What I started out to say was that next week I would answer any questions in your letters and make appropriate comments on bits of news etc. It is nice to know that my letters have started reaching you, sort of as though I had tossed a string to you, one of those colored paper ones that you throw from a ship when you sail, and you had reached out and caught the end of my colored piece of paper. A frail connection, in some ways, but at least a connection.

This letter will be a poor attempt to tell you about my New Year's weekend in Davos. A poor attempt, because it is impossible, for many reasons, to put on paper all that we did and saw and heard and felt. A colored movie camera, constantly with us, would have been the only way to capture it all, and then even that would have left out our personal reactions to various episodes, and it is often one's reaction that makes the difference between an ordinary occurrence and an extremely interesting or amusing event.

One of the recently arrived clerks, a girl named Cordelia Dodson, was persuaded to go with me (although I must admit that I didn't have to do very much persuading). Friday night I moved from my temporary flat into Betty's, so it was late when I got to bed and the strange quarters prevented me from sleeping too well. [Church bells outside my bedroom window rang every quarter hour and contributed to my restless sleep. It took me weeks to get used to them.]

We sleepily found our train and sat in silence for some time, not feeling very sociable at that hour. But about eight o'clock we woke up enough to lurch to the dining car for breakfast. It was the first time I had been in a dining car for about three years, I think, and I was properly thrilled. Even though the coffee was almost as bad as that I had made for myself. We were joined by a Greek internee dressed in British battle dress, who talked to us in a steady stream in what he fondly imagined was English, but due to the low tone of voice in which he spoke and the paucity of his vocabulary and the originality of his pronunciation, we neither of us understood more than a dozen words. And he refused, of course, to speak either French or German. But he was very pleasant, insisted on paying for our breakfast, waited for us when we changed trains in Zurich and carried our bags to the other train, and then dragged off his gloves, solemnly shook hands with us and then snapped into the quivering British salute. By that time we were giggling so hard that it was difficult to compose our faces sufficiently to be polite to him.

Third-class carriages were too crowded, so we splurged and went into a second-class. The scenery was still fairly uninteresting, although we went along the edge of the lake for a long time and towards the end of it caught glimpses of snow covered mountains. We changed again at Landquart and from then on were so excited by the views that we stood in the corridor in order to see better. We got to Davos Platz shortly after one o'clock and, to our great pleasure, were met by a sleigh from the hotel where we had made reservations through a travel bureau here in Bern. We climbed up on the high seat, were snugly tucked in with a bearskin rug, our baggage was put on a sled behind, and off we went with bells jingling and the clop clop of the horses' hooves on the hard snow beating out the time. We were both so thrilled we practically fell out, trying to see everything at once. It was a clear sunny day, very cold, and the air almost intoxicating. Along the road were rows of trees with big heavy clusters of red berries, each bunch capped with a thick layer of snow. Most effective, the red and white together that way. We saw no cars, only the sleighs and people on foot and on skis. It seems to me that here children ski before they are old enough to walk, but I suppose not. All the clothes are gay and bright and look like travel posters or fashion advertisements. And the people look gay too, and happy. I didn't see any of the sanatorium patients, of which there are still so many.

Our arrival at the hotel kept up the reputation of Swiss hospitality, for the manager and his assistant were on the steps to greet us as we drove up, and the assistant personally took us to our rooms. Then, still in ski clothes, of course, we came down for a very nice meal in the dining room. By the time we were through, it was almost three and it seemed silly to start skiing that afternoon. (Both of us had been warned that if we broke a leg or an arm up there, that when we returned we would also have our necks broken. The Boss echoes verbatim all your warnings about the danger of the conjunction of slippery wooden sticks and slippery snow.)

And anyway we had a couple of errands to do, like buying mittens, and we wanted to explore the town. We got some pretty knitted and leather mittens, went down to the skating rink for a while to watch even younger children twirl expertly on the ice and then wandered back to find out what time the *funicular* [cablecar] went up the mountain in the morning.

While we were reading the poster an apologetic youngster in Army clothes approached us and timidly asked us if we were Americans or English. He had followed us a couple of blocks, listening to us and trying to make up his mind. We assured him we were American and from that time on our social life in Davos was guaranteed a success. He took us into the nearby bar that is the center of American life in Davos and where you can go in the morning for coffee, stay all day if you want, playing bridge, have tea and cakes in the afternoon, and so on. The couple that run it are most *simpático* and of course financial wizards as they must be to keep straight the confusion of charging and treating and paying back that goes on every day. The boys keep their sugar, which they got from the Red Cross, there on a shelf, and Anne, the girl, brings it down for them whenever they order coffee.

It wasn't long before we were completely surrounded by American boys, all incredulous of the fact that we were really Americans. [The boys were all internees, of course, military men who had reached the safety of neutral Switzerland by various routes and told hair-raising stories.] It reminded me of those two nights when I played at being a Clubmobile girl [in North Africa] and talked to those boys who had not seen a white girl for eight months, much less an American. They are just starved for news from home and for conversation with someone who really understands what they mean. It really is a little pathetic.

I was amazed at the number of New Englanders. My own pet, an attractive dark-haired fellow named Sam (gave me a queer feeling at first, I have known so few), came from Connecticut and was more intelligent and better educated, as well as older, than most. Cordelia's most constant escort was a lad called Junior, scarcely 19 years old and had been in the Army two years. But a precocious 19, I must say, and a charming youngster. Cordelia complained that she was getting them younger and younger; her first date in Bern was 24 (she is 29). On the train coming back she was "picked up" by an earnest 16-year-old.

Sam and Junior of course took us to the train in a sleigh, and we had great difficulty persuading them that the Swiss would take an awfully dim view of their accompanying us to Bern. They are not allowed to leave the town, you see. And one of their favorite forms of amusement is to spend half an hour at the station just as a train is leaving, pretending to try to avoid and evade the guards. The poor guards are driven half crazy by them. But this time, no matter how loudly they announced that they were leaving with us, the guards refused to pay any attention to them, much to their disappointment. We had to promise and cross our hearts that we would come up again soon—which I hope we can do.

You can well imagine that I had no trouble sleeping when I finally got home. Even the quarter hour chimes on the church outside my window had no effect on me.

10 January 1945

Dear Mother and Father:

The apartment is just as nice as I hoped it would be, and I feel completely justified in forgoing the convenience of a bathtub for the charm and delightfulness of the place. As I think I told you, Betty [who was leaving to get married] has lived there for almost two years and before that her brother and for part of the time, his wife, lived there. There is a long hall, with the "bathroom" at one end near the front door, then at the other end of the hall are my two rooms. In between the windows look out into an inner courtyard and chimney pots and clothes lines and balconies. I shall try to get a picture of it some day. Part of the first room is cur-tained off and has a small sink, a gas water heater (which I never use) and a table with a two-burner gas stove on it. And another table that had a series of shelves on it. I promptly took the shelves off and put them on the floor, thereby making it possible for me to reach the top shelf which previously had been too high, and clearing off the table so that I could eat there. I bought some pretty blue and white and yellow oil cloth at the local equivalent of the 5-and-10 and covered the table with it, moved in my electric heater, took down the old rather dingy curtains and put up yards and yards of blue and white checked gingham and now my "kitchen" is almost the nicest part of the flat.

Outside the curtained-off space is what could be the dining room, with a large table, a dresser that I covered with a red and white checked table cloth and decorated with a basket of apples, and the big tile stove. The two little old ladies who own the place light the big stove every morning and it keeps warm all day. And my pet discovery, which I read about in the Martha Albrand book, is that apples put in the oven part of stoves like this fill the air with a wonderful smell and after about four days one has delicious baked apples. They are awfully good as hand-warmers too, when one has just come in from the cold. Just reach into my oven and take out a warm apple to hold for a few minutes and smell from time to time.

The room beyond is the bed-sitting room, but I must admit that I use it more as a bedroom than as a sitting room. There is a smaller stove in here, but usually I feel it is too much trouble to light it and it takes too long to heat the room. There is also a fireplace but I have not tried it yet. Wood is pretty hard to get and I shall save the fireplace for special occasions.

Betty left me her radio, which is a very good one. And I bought two plants, some kind of *primavera* I think. And soon I shall get a new couch cover, meanwhile my red plaid blanket [from North Africa] brightens up the room [as it brightens our present living room in Cambridge]. It is really a nice room, the windows look out practically into a bell tower and one can see a glimpse of the river below and the hills beyond. In the spring and summer I expect to use the room much more, when there is no heating problem.

I had my housewarming last Sunday afternoon and am told it was a very pleasant party. Ice is hard to buy here, for some reason, so I solved the problem by putting a big pan out the window overnight, and there I had all the ice I needed! My icebox is the wide window ledge between the inner and the outer windows and things stay just cold enough there without freezing. Someday I will send you part of my ration card, so that you can see how much we are allowed every month. It can be done, but it takes careful thinking.

Yesterday morning on the way to the office I discovered a new outdoors market. Apparently on Tuesdays the street next to me becomes a big meat market. Yesterday it was snowing hard in the morning and it was really quite a sight, the canvas-topped booths, the softly falling snow and the tremendous array of whole sides of beef, hearts, kidneys, brain, pigs' feet, dozens of different kinds of sausages, and other things to which I could not put a name. What I cannot understand is how, with the limited coupon allowance for meat, all that could ever be bought. Maybe the restaurants and hotels do their shopping there.

Thanks for the kind words to the Boss [possibly in a Christmas card]. But then you are a bit prejudiced.

19 January 1945

Dear Mother and Father:

We went to a concert of Slavic music the other night. Not too good, the orchestra was not integrated and both the conductor and the musicians were hampered by Teutonic stolidity, which is not helpful in interpreting Slavic music. They ended with the *1812 Overture*, which I had last heard in Italy, and the contrast was amazing. In Italy the orchestra was completely carried away by it, and so was the audience, and they had to give three encores of the last part. Here the audience seemed apathetic in comparison. Next week I am going to hear a Bach program for one, two, three and four pianos. I will be interested to see if that is better.

Someday I must settle down and take some conventional French lessons. My present vocabulary is the most curious hodgepodge of words. In North Africa I learned medical terms and words like those for kerosene lamps, feather pillows and other things that we bought for our tent housekeeping. Here I am keeping house in French, not only my own but the Boss's too. I pay all his bills and give his domestics the necessary instructions as to how many for dinner, etc. And then there is my own shopping. One can read the word for turnip a dozen times and not remember it, but when one has to go and buy the things, the word becomes fixed in one's memory. It really is fun and I am trying to be as independent as I can, even though sometimes I have to force myself to enter a store. You know, in spite of everything, fundamentally I am really quite shy and unsure of myself. But I have discovered that success in such cases consists in fooling the largest number of people most of the time. And usually one fools oneself too. So it is only in moments of soul-searching that I realize that what I really am and what I seem to be are two quite different things. However, as time goes on, I think that they are getting more alike rather than farther apart.

All this about turnips arose from the fact that I decided to have an Irish stew this weekend, and started my shopping for it this morning. I'll let you know how it comes out. Back at Rollins Place [where I had lived in Boston] I used to make a very good stew but I may have lost my hand at those things.

26 January 1945

Dear Mother and Father:

Wonder if I will ever outgrow my love of snowy weather. A slight snowstorm and I feel like a six-year-old, and when

one gets continual snow as one does here—well, I am in a
perpetual flurry of delight. It has been snowing off and on
for a week now, and Bern is lovely. From time to time it
clears up a little and some of the snow in the streets melts off
and one gets a brief and tantalizing glimpse of the mountains
to the east, but most of the time the skies are gray and the
big white flakes drift softly down. This morning it was
almost a blizzard as I walked to work, and I arrived looking
like a snow maiden covered with snow from head to foot and
with a foolish grin on my face. I looked so happy and people
are so friendly when it is snowing, that everyone smiled back
at me, a priest lifted his hat to me and a cheery Swiss peas-
ant grinned at me and murmured *"Lustig, eh?"* as he passed.
It is almost lunchtime now and it is still snowing hard—
guess I had better dust off my new skis and ski to town for
lunch!

Before I forget it, from now on my monthly cheque will
be $100 instead of $102 or whatever it was. There has been a
terrible confusion about my salary, which I don't believe will
be settled until I can do it in person. According to the latest
instructions, I received a so-called raise, which amounts to
$500 less a year than I received at my last post! Figure that
out, if you can! (The Boss said, "Huh, supporting your
father now?")

I have given up and am satisfied as long as my allotment
home is uninterrupted and as long as I get enough here to
live on according to the luxury to which I am now becoming
accustomed—and as long as they don't make that "raise" (sic)
retroactive. What worries me is how I am ever going to
come down to the level of a $20-a-week job [my pre-war
wage] after the war. My standards of living are so much
above that now. What with my maid at my last post and
wool gabardine dresses from Peck & Peck—guess I had better get married and let someone else worry about paying my
bills!

You will be glad to know that we talked to [Mrs. Dulles]

the mother of the Little Princesses [as I had called the Dulles girls in the 1920s] this morning and I hope to see her in a couple of weeks.

I am keeping the Boss supplied with tidbits of one sort or another. Yesterday it was a paragraph from Father's letter and today it was a piece of maple sugar. I hope to get him in the purring stage soon. Seriously, as time goes by I am enjoying this job and working with him more and more. The job seems to have the unusual quality of expanding and growing as the people in it expand and grow. So many jobs present a challenge for the first couple of weeks, but then as things become routine, the job itself becomes routine and becomes dull and uninteresting. But this one, *enfin*, really seems to unfold as one progresses and new views and vistas are opened as one goes down the path (whoops, when did I start that figure of flowery speech?). But I think you know what I mean. To be brief, I am really quite content here. (Remind me of that six months from now, will you?)

As far as letters are concerned, this has been a wonderful week, with all sorts of old friends turning up for the first time in years; there was a very welcome one from Marty Fenn, my junior year roommate at Stanford, and a lovely long one from my inattentive godfather, Feg Bartter who is in Guatemala with the Pan American Health Service. [Dr. Frederick Bartter, a resident at Mass General, had been my godfather when I was baptized and confirmed in 1940 at the Church of the Advent in Boston. He took his responsibilities quite seriously as I was so new to the Christian faith.] Didn't I do well? Then two from Mother and one from Father, three *New Yorkers*, two *New York Times* and wonder of wonders a package from Richard with a couple of pounds of coffee! He is a lamb, and you have no idea how welcome that is. Even when I add chicory to mine (makes better *cafe au lait*, really) the monthly ration here is scarcely enough to last a week. So that which is coming from you will receive just as enthusiastic a welcome, and I wish you would send more, if it doesn't cut off your own ration. Is it still rationed at home? If it is, please don't send anymore—but if it is not, I would love a couple of more pounds. I gave Mildred, in spite of her protests, about a third of what Richard sent me, because I knew that some was coming from you. I use about a pound a month, I guess, if I eat all my breakfasts home, as I prefer doing. I shall try to buy a coffee grinder tomorrow, if I am successful I shall let you know. Otherwise it is easier to receive it already ground.

I am now the proud possessor of a five-pound can of egg powder which one of my friends here sold me from some he got from the States four years ago. I hope it is still good— my mouth is watering at the thought of soufflés, scrambled eggs and omelettes and such.

Finally got around to eating snails the other night. Very good they were too. Wonder what there is left for me now, I have eaten octopus in Italy, squid in its own ink in Spain and snails in Switzerland. Of course, there is still bird's nest soup in China. Or shall I settle first for elevenses in Chocorua? I think maybe yes. [Longfellow's "pause in the day's occupation" came at the end of the day "between the dark and the daylight," but it was our family's custom to pause in mid-morning for coffee and Mother's homemade bread. Often Father would read aloud from Dornford Yates, one of our favorite British authors—not exactly a "children's hour" but a very important custom for nurturing family togetherness.]

Last Sunday was one of those nice days that come all too seldom. The Boss was away but it was my Sunday to work and I had a lot of back filing to do, so I thought I would come in anyway for a couple of hours. I slept late, had a leisurely breakfast and washed some clothes, then wandered to the office and leisurely did what needed to be done (that in itself was a treat, as leisure in the office is rare), then home again for a long afternoon listening to the symphony on the radio, keeping warm by my little woodstove and reading Galsworthy. Did I tell you that I am reading *Forsyte Saga* for the first time, having started it at least a dozen times in the past, and enjoying it tremendously. Particularly after my recent stay in London. I use a map of London as a bookmark and look up their walks and wanderings from time to time.

In between chapters I made my now famous Irish stew. It was a huge success and the titillating odor of gently simmering lamb and celery roots and carrots and turnips and onions filled the apartment, blending deliciously with the fragrance of the apples in my oven and the faint smell of wood smoke from my fire. The clock in the church tower outside chimed the quarter hours, the wood crackled in the stove, a mouse ran scrambling across the attic floor above and the snow brushed softly against the windowpane. I almost resented the intrusion of my "date" for the evening when he came for me after supper (Irish stew, of course, with a glass of milk and baked apple for dessert). I used only 300 grams of lamb for the stew and got three big meals off it, which I think is pretty good. And if I didn't eat so much, I would have had four or five meals off it.

With Sundays like that *"chez moi"* I don't mind at all having to stay in Berne (without the "e" officially, but I prefer it with) to do a little work every other Sunday.

I don't believe I was properly appreciative of the tremendous sacrifice involved in saving those little packages of sugar for me. I realize what it must have meant to you, and am deeply grateful. Imagine, both stealing *and* doing without sugar in your coffee!!!

You have no idea how many people get pleasure from my magazines and newspapers. Me of course, then others in the office and the legation in general and when everyone in Berne is through with them I alternate sending them to my friends among the internees. And you can imagine how they appreciate them. (My Red Cross training coming through, I am thinking of asking for a small salary from the Red Cross, since I still seem to be doing work for them.) It was good to get news of Paul M, Ted R and Col. S [people I knew in

Madrid] and your version of their inquiries was very ego-inflating. I am glad that I am beginning to create my own light instead of shining in reflected glory! Paul M was always a favorite of mine. As soon as spring comes I expect to spend many weekends in and near Geneva, and I shall look up Mr. Squire then.

3 February 1945

Dear Mother and Father:

The concert last night was very good—I am enclosing the program to pad out the letter and for Father's edification. Fischer [probably the classical pianist Edwin Fischer] has often played in the states, so you have probably heard him play. He is a fascinating person to watch, with a great shock of white hair that he tosses about. He conducts the orchestra from the piano and gets tremendously excited about the whole thing, so even if one cannot see his hands on the keys, the performance is visually satisfying.

I hope to get to Geneva this weekend. I've got a dinner date there, and I want to take a bath!

10 February 1945

Dear Mother and Father:

The telephone man came to make my telephone ring more loudly, as I discovered that I didn't hear it at night. One of my beaus has taken to calling me about 12:30, a habit which I must discourage, but at least it served the purpose of showing me that the telephone did me no good at all after I am asleep. Anyway, the telephone man spoke almost no French and I speak almost no German, so at times things were a little confused. And then I was still in bed when he arrived, and I find it a little hard to maintain my usual poise with my hair up in bobby pins and dressed in pajamas and bathrobe. But we finally got it fixed and it makes enough noise to wake the people in the next apartment below.

Last weekend I finally got to Geneva, but as I couldn't leave here until the end of the afternoon, the trip down was made after dark and I saw nothing of the country. And then Sunday was foggy and rainy, so most of my sightseeing was confined to the nightclubs on Saturday night. But that was fun and my escort was a New Hampshire man, a Dartmouth graduate.

So you can see that we had a lot in common. I'll tell you more about him some other time.

16 February 1945

Dear Mother and Father:

I have treated you very badly for two weeks now for which I am very sorry. The first short letter I couldn't help, but last week not only was I busy but in a bad humor and I took it out in my letter, I am afraid. So this week I am starting on Friday, to see if I can get caught up on some of the things I want to say.

First a bit of bragging. Yesterday the Boss said he hoped to get another stenographer soon, which would relieve me of most of the dictation, as he wanted me to be sort of an executive secretary or office manager! I am rather pleased, not only because it is the sort of job I prefer, but also at the implied satisfaction with my work or something. I shall now forgive him that Christmas cable! He meant well by it but it was too effusive to be consistent with the length of time I had been here or with any thoughtful evaluation of my abilities or capabilities.

Madam [Dulles] arrived the first of the week. As yet I have not had a chance to see her, but I wrote her a note when she first got here, asking her to let me know if there was anything I could do for her, and then Mildred and I sent her a "garden bowl," a charming earthenware bowl planted with snowdrops, crocus, grape, hyacinth and ferns. I had a nice note in return from her and hope to see her soon.

The week was a busy one, the Boss was away part of the time and getting him off was a hectic business. And my social calendar was well filled with lunch dates, dinner dates and cocktail dates almost every day. While I am not exactly the belle of Berne, I seem to have an adequate supply of friends who like to do things with me. Mostly I enjoy it, but every once in a while I get a "sawdust in my mouth feeling" about the whole thing and stay home and read Galsworthy for a few nights. I suppose it is because, as Feg Bartter said, "one is trying to grow roots in the sand" and subconsciously one realizes that these are all shipboard acquaintances. (Mixed metaphor, but you know what I mean.)

One of my dates was a movie one and we went to see *Bambi*, which I had somehow missed before. I was enchanted by it, parts are really very well done. It is fun what memories I am accumulating, the autumn leaves reminded me of that lovely walk up Puck Street with Jessie Aiken. And on the way home I suddenly got hungry for some cinnamon toast and remembered the wonderful cinnamon toast that we used to make when we were waiting outside Bizerte to go to Italy. Supper used to be at five and by nine we were all hungry again, so Buff brought her can of cinnamon and the rest of us contributed bouillon cubes or bread swiped from the mess or butter likewise—nothing ever tasted so good, eight or ten of us crowded together on the two cots in the little tent.

Have I told you about the wooden-soled shoes the children wear here much to their delight as they can make so much noise walking down the street? And about the rawhide school bags they wear strapped to their backs? And about the dogs that draw the milk carts, and the sleighs that deliver things in snowy weather and the piles of snow on the overhanging eaves that they have to shovel off every once in a while? And the big bunches of white lilac in the florist windows now, and the bright mimosa?

24 February 1945

Dear Mother and Father:

For some reason which I have as yet been unable to determine, probably because I felt that what with only eleven

228

hours a day at the office and doing my own housekeeping (at least to the extent of most of my laundry, my marketing and my cooking), and trying to get some reading and letter writing done in between times, I really did not have enough to do—I am now taking Italian lessons twice a week! Thoroughly frivolous, because they don't speak even a *patois* of Italian in this part of Switzerland, but I get so tired of having a useful reason for everything I do that it is almost recreation to study a language I don't need. It really is fun; Cordelia and I are doing it together during our lunch hours Wednesday and Friday, and our teacher is a very young, very charming Italian internee who works at the Italian air attaché's office. He is very serious about teaching us, wants English lessons in return (which we told him we would be too busy to give him), and now he refuses any money and says he does it for the pleasure of it!? He comes from Milano and has been here in Switzerland with his wife for over a year now. I am amazed at how quickly the little I learned when I was in Italy is coming back to me, and already after two lessons I am way ahead of Cordelia. He won't let us talk anything but Italian during our lesson period—the result is sometimes a long silence! It is good for my French too, because that is our most common language and before and after class we talk French together.

Hearing Italian again makes me almost homesick for the three months I was there, for Mike's Place where Doug and I ate so often and for the Italian family I stayed with when I went up to visit him. Maybe that is one reason I wanted to study it again, as it reminds me of so many pleasant things. And another reason could be that I would like to come home that way, when I finally do get around to coming home.

I had the pleasure of meeting Mrs. D. a few days ago, and was completely charmed. She is quite different from what I had imagined, although I am not quite sure what I expected. I hope that I can see something of her from time to time.

I also met the minister [deputy chief of mission at the

embassy] today for the first time. He seems most pleasant and conveyed your greetings to me. I really should by this time be used to people saying they had recently lunched or dined with my family, but I still have been unable to find the proper response and just grin in a pleased way. There should be a suitable answer, but it leaves me with the same feeling as when people say to a child "My, how you've grown!"

Finally one of my suitcases has arrived from my last post. Peg has promised the other one by train in the near future. You have no idea how glad I was to see it, as it had many things I have needed for months in it, like my gray flannel skirt and jacket and towels and sheets. The Swiss idea of cleanliness is two clean sheets every four or five weeks! Even after my "no sheet and Army blanket" existence that seems dirty to me, but now I have my own sheets and can have clean ones as often as I want. My two little old ladies will probably think it is another one of those crazy American ideas, but should be glad as it will save them even the monthly laundering of the sheets they provided me with before.

Last weekend was my out-of-town weekend and I went to Gstaad on Saturday evening with some friends including a British couple named Leslie, Don and Jerry M. We stopped off at our black-market restaurant for another one of those oh-so-high teas that I described to you once before, and then persuaded the charming girl who helps run the place, to come skiing with us. She speaks some English, having spent eight months in England before the war, and is a most attractive person.

In Berne the weather had been warm and spring-like, with all vestiges of snow quite melted away, except for a gray patch or two down by the river. But as we got up into the mountains, although it didn't get much colder, there was plenty of snow on the ground. And what excited me most of all were the covered bridges. I just hadn't happened to see any before, and we must have passed by or through a good

230

dozen on our way to Gstaad. It was too dark to get a picture, much as I wanted to.

No weekend would be complete without my bath, so I rang for the maid the next morning to draw one for me. Lovely, luxurious feeling to relax in a tub of hot water. Except that this tub, one of those high ones with feet, wobbled in a most disconcerting manner. Almost made one seasick. I think that the fourth volume of my book will be called "Bathing in Switzerland or Bathtubs I Have Known." [I wonder what I had in mind for the first three volumes.] You, Mother, may be able to remember Swiss hotels by the toilet paper, but I shall recall them by their tubs.

We all met for breakfast and then drove back towards Saanenmoser to the station to which we had shipped our skis. I was a little loath to attempt the ski lift to the top of the mountain but allowed myself to be persuaded by Don, who said he would "look after" me. I should have known better. For when we got to the top the run down was obviously too icy for me. So Don agreed to meet me at the other lift on the other side of the peak in about forty minutes. Being a well brought up young lady and accustomed to people who take their *rendez-vous* seriously, I really expected to meet him there. I took some pictures and laboriously wandered over to the other side of the mountain, carrying my skis most of the way, feeling that in this case with a steep drop on one side of the foot-wide path, discretion was the better part of valor. Well, to make a long story short, I met them three and half hours later at the hotel at Saanenmoser! I, of course, had waited most of that time by the ski lift, thinking that if they didn't find me there they would worry, knowing that I was a novice skier. But what with one thing and another, they had made another run down to the hotel and then it was lunchtime and the line for the *funi* [funicular] was so long, that they decided to eat there. Edge Leslie had also expected to meet them on top, so he and I eventually joined forces and after looking once more for them, skied down. He sort of chaperoned me over the steep places, and for the first time I really got the feeling of skiing. The sun had warmed the snow by this time, the slopes were wide and open, and I traversed back and forth with the wind and sun in my face, so pleased with myself that I almost started yodeling. It was lovely.

At the halfway house, I decided to take the *funi* the rest of the way down, as the lower half of the run was still icy and as I had never ridden in a *funi* like that. We met Nancy Leslie at the bottom, she hadn't skied at all (she is the one who skied with me that day at Wengen when we sat in the sun all day) and she told us where the others were. Jerry had to rush back to Berne, so I got no lunch at all. Needless to say, I was a little annoyed by the whole thing. Knowing how indefinite one's plans are when skiing, it would never have occurred to me to make plans to meet during the day, but Don had been so insistent that I agreed. I suppose I am the "boy who stood on the burning deck" sort of a person, but that is partly your fault. I think that I shall bring my children up to be always late for meeting people, and to change their plans if it so suits them without telling anyone. It will save them a lot of wear and tear.

My home address is Kramgasse 6. A lot of my shopping is done on the Kramgasse now. As I walk up towards the Zeitglocke, on the right hand side just before I get to the Zeitglocke is the bakery where I buy the best bread in town, called "English Toast." I go in and say *"Ein English Toast, bitte. Merci."* Which is perfectly correct albeit a little silly-sounding. The patisserie is on the corner of Luisenstrasse and Thunstrasse. My dairy is on the Marktgasse on the left hand side just beyond the Zeitglocke. The vegetable stand where I buy endive almost every day (and to think that once I wouldn't eat it) is also on the Kramgasse near the bakery.

Sometime I will try to draw you a picture of the stove. It is just a big box made out of brown and white tiles. At one end is the door for the wood and another for the draft, and

232

in one side is another little door which opens into a small tile-lined hole, which is the oven where I bake the apples. It never gets terribly hot, one couldn't do bread, except perhaps if one built up a big roaring fire.

3 March 1945

Dear Mother and Father:

This has been another one of those weeks and the length of this letter depends on how early the Boss gets in. He was laid up with the gout for two days, which meant I spent most of the time running back and forth between here and his house. Good exercise but not conducive to a smoothly running office. And then I am the proud owner of a lovely new safe with drawers like a filing cabinet inside, and of course I had to take this week to try to re-arrange my files. And then twice this week I had to get up at the crack of dawn to come to the office and give some packages to some people who were taking an early train. So you can see that I have not been idle.

One of those early morning jaunts was really quite fun. I had been almost ordered not to do it, as the Boss said that I had enough to do. But there wasn't anyone else to do it and no good alternative, so I figured that what he didn't know wouldn't hurt him, and set my alarm for 5:30! A taxi was waiting outside my door at 6 and in the apparently middle of the night I came up to the office, got the stuff and went down to the station. It was my New England friend who was leaving and we had a pleasant, albeit sleepy breakfast in the Bahnhof Buffet before he took his train. Then, as it was only 7 o'clock, I decided to walk leisurely back to the office. Night was just being chased over the western hills and as I walked across the bridge, I was almost breathless with the beauty of the early morning. In the east, a little to my left, the jagged peaks of the mountains were dark against an incredible robin's egg blue sky. Further to the east the horizon was streaked with salmon pink. Below the bridge the river lay as calm as a millpond, reflecting the colors of the sky and the dark bare trees along the bank and a puff of smoke from a house on the other side. The birds were just waking and trying out their morning voices. To my right, upstream, the valley was still blurred with wisps of fog and mist and the streetlights going up the side of the hill looked like a necklace of gold beads hanging in midair. And to finish off the picture, the full moon, looking almost translucent in the growing daylight, rested just above the Moorish-looking domes of the Bundeshaus.

I floated rather than walked the rest of the way up the street and it took the practicalness of a hot bath to bring me back down to earth. I have decided that that is the best way of solving this bath problem of mine, especially since our gas ration is now so low that I daren't heat water at home to wash in. There is a lovely big bathtub here at the office and plenty of hot water, so I shall either come in early a couple of times a week, or the nights that I work late I shall stay even later and take a bath.

Last Sunday the Boss was away. It was my Sunday to work, so I put in an appearance for a couple of hours and then Emmy [a Dulles family friend] and Mrs. D and I went out to lunch together. Emmy is a delightful person; she rather wants me to share an apartment with her, but I think that would be a mistake. I am liking my living alone too much. She seems to have heard a lot about me, and fortunately doesn't seem to be disappointed in the actuality. She wrote to her secretary that I was always laughing. . . .

The first part of an exceptionally long letter dated 8 March 1945 was mostly about letters received, including one from Doug after an eight-month gap due entirely to letters lost or misdirected. Having shared my excitement and pleasure and anxiety over that situation, I then went on to write about some of my experiences the previous weekend:

Last Saturday I got in as usual practically at the crack of dawn, and found a friend of mine from the consulate in Lugano in ahead of me, pacing the floor of the office. He had to drive to Lugano that day with a newly repaired car, and the friend that was supposed to drive with him had been detained elsewhere. So he was faced with the prospect of a day's drive alone, partly over snowy roads. Just in fun I offered to go with him, but told him that I couldn't leave until lunchtime, as it was my weekend off but I had to work all morning. And I didn't think the matter justified my asking for the extra time. But he thought it did, so as soon as the Boss came in he asked if I might go. And much to my surprise the Boss said I might! (It turned out later that he thought there might be some mail I might bring back on Sunday, but there wasn't.) So in a flurry of excitement I told Mildred where everything was. (Fortunately I had been a good girl and had transcribed the dictation he had given me late the night before, and fortunately I had just finished my letter to you—that breathless bit at the end was done just as the Boss arrived). So with a minimum of delay I was ready. We drove to my apartment to pick up my toothbrush and pyjamas and get some socks as the Boss very paternally insisted I should be warmly dressed for the mountain part of the trip, and left Berne at 10:30. I was so journey-proud that it was all I could do to sit still in the car.

As far as Luzern the weather continued nice and the country was lovely to drive through. Snowy mountains in the distance and the nearer hills brown-green as they hesitated between winter and spring. There was even a softness about the bare branches of the trees, as if their sharp winter outlines were being blurred by the warmth of the sun. I saw many of my favorite covered bridges and we drove through many picturesque little villages, each one looking just like an impossible tourist postcard or like a child's toy. The heavy overhanging eaves, the long sloping roofs of either red tile or weathered wooden shingles, the carved gingerbread decorations and balconies—it is almost too picturesque, you don't feel that there is any reality to it.

We had lunch in Luzern in the Holbeinstube where, theoretically, Holbein used to work or eat or something. And we drove through William Tell's town with a big statue of him in the main square. It was fun to see the difference in atmosphere and architecture and even people in different cantons. Partly it is the difference between Protestant and Catholic communities—Don and I decided that a Catholic country or canton is much more *simpático* than a Protestant, at least a German Protestant!

There was too much snow for us to go over the mountains all the way by car, but we drove up to Göschenen and took the train there, having first put the car on a flat freight car. Even driving up that far, we had trouble with the snow and got stuck twice, *grâce à* a fair blond German who got stuck ahead of us. First we pushed him out and then he had to push us out. There were signs of many avalanches down the mountainsides and we were both a little relieved when we got safely to Göschenen. Through the Gotthard tunnel took only fifteen minutes and we came out on the other side into an Italian spring [of the Ticino Canton]. Really, it is just like a different country—the day had clouded up on the Luzern side and was gray and cold, but on the Lugano side the sun was shining, the sky blue, the grass beginning to get green.

Sorry, but it is now Saturday noon and I've been too hectic to finish this. Continued in my next.

16 March 1945

Dear Mother and Father:

Where did I leave you so suddenly last week? Just as I came through the Gotthard tunnel, I think, out into the warm Swiss-Italian spring. As I said before, it was amazing how the countryside itself changed and became Italian in character rather than Swiss. The drive down into the valley was lovely and Don amused me with tales of the odd characters who live in Lugano, which seems to be the center of eccentricity as Florence used to be. There were the two little old ladies who lived together up on top of a hill, having run away from their families forty years before. And the girl who keeps snakes and rides the street cars with them around her neck. And the widow who had her husband pickled and is mad at the Swiss because they won't let her keep him in the parlor of her house. And the man who believes in the art of dinner conversation so strongly that even when he eats by himself, he keeps up a scintillating conversation with himself. Don kept me in giggles all the way down. Then he told me about the little town he used to live in, where their house was partway up a hill from the village and on top of the hill was a shrine which the villagers built one year when there were heavy early snows and their vineyards were in danger. So they took the statue of the Madonna out of their little church and carried it up the hill to the edge of the snow, and the Madonna lifted her hands and the snow stopped and the grapes were saved. Every year there is a procession up to the shrine and the path went right through Don's yard and past his house. So he and his wife gave a party for the whole village every year, when they came back down the hill. And the villagers used to leave presents for them, but it was not good form to hand them to their host and hostess, so they would tuck them in odd places around the house and for weeks afterwards Don and his wife would find a couple of eggs in a vase or a few apples behind a cushion or a jar of jelly under a chair.

The medieval walled town of Bellinzona lies in the mountain end of a long green fertile valley with Locarno at the other end. Parts of the old walls still stand and there is a fairy-book castle on a hill in the middle of the town. Next time I hope to get some pictures, or some postcards at least. It reminded me a little of Avila and when one was on the valley side it was interesting to look back and see how the walls in front and the mountains behind made an impregnable fortress out of it. The valley was a pretty one, many vineyards with stone walls around them and the vines supported on stone posts. There were little stone shrines along the road, church spires out of the huddle of roofs of each little village, lots of gay and rather dirty little children playing in the streets—all quite different from the clean orderliness of German Swiss towns.

We drove into Lugano just at twilight, with a bit of sunset color still in the sky and reflected in the lake. The evening star had just come out and across the water lights came on one by one, except for a big dark patch in the middle that was blacked-out Italy. I even got into Italy: just for the fun of it we drove across the bridge and into Campione, which of course is liberated Italy, surrounded by Switzerland on all sides. It was too dark to see the town, but I got a kick out it anyway. Then I met some friends for dinner and finally got back to my hotel, the Walter, right on the lakefront. The bed was big and comfortable, the stars were bright and a gentle breeze made the water lap softly against the shore. It didn't take long for me to get to sleep.

I had intended to sleep late the next morning, but the day was so bright and sunny and the birds made so much noise, that I gave it up about eight o'clock and ordered my bath drawn. Then I had breakfast sent up and sat on my balcony in the sun, in just a skirt and blouse! I love the winter and the snow, but it is so nice when spring comes again.

After breakfast I "did" the town, almost from one end to the other, along the lakefront watching the fishing boats, up and down the arcade streets, and even partway up San Salvatore. During part of the morning I was theoretically taking a large police dog for a walk, but it is nearer the truth to say that the large police dog took me for a walk. To make it more complicated, the dog spoke only French, and, it being a very large dog, I often lost the argument of which way we would go. I flew along in his wake across flower beds and lawns that were plainly posted "do not walk on the grass" or whatever it is they say in Italian, up stairs, around lamp

238

posts, and for three glorious minutes while we chased lizards along a stone wall where they had been peacefully slumbering in the sun. I was exhausted by the time I persuaded him to go back to the consulate with me. My lunch date took me to a *Tessinois* restaurant and afterward drove me around, down along the lake to the barbed-wire barricade in front of the tunnel to the Italian border, and up to the top of Monte Bre. The flowers were just beginning to come out, yellow primroses and blue periwinkles and lavender violets hidden in the grass. (Out my window today I can see snowdrops and crocus in the backyard). The view from the top of Monte Bre was breathtaking. It is supposed to be the sunniest place in Switzerland.

The trip back was enlivened only by the Elizabeth Goudge book I had to read, by the conductor who spotted me as a foreigner without my even opening my mouth and thereafter when he stuck his head in the door to announce anything, he would do it in French, German and Italian for the benefit of the others in the compartment, then turn to me and with a bow repeat it all in English. It was most amusing.

There was quite a blizzard at the top of the San Gotthardt and I thought what fun if we got stuck there. But we didn't and I uneventfully reached home by elevenish, full of determination to go back to Lugano at the first opportunity.

Saturday morning

The following week was jammed with work and social engagements. Don Bigelow's wife arrived and they gave a big cocktail party, our Steak Club had a meeting, a delightful English friend and former colleague of Richard's turned up and we lunched together and I learned that he [Richard] was planning to go home soon. Two new secretaries arrived and I had to ease them into the routine and into life in Berne for neither of them speak either French or German! (My strongest emotion was that of sympathetic pity for Betty and

Mildred; if I was as full of helpful hints and criticisms my first weeks here, I don't see how they stood it.) Two packages arrived Thursday, one with books and the other with coffee, cigarettes etc. Please thank your friend again, Father, and tell him that I am more convinced than ever of their superiority. Thank you too.

Sunday I went skiing at Saanenmoser again, with John, Van and one of the new girls. It was again an incredibly beautiful day and there had been a meter of new snow. I am improving tremendously and made one run from the halfway house to the bottom without falling once! Which is impressive when I realized that probably I haven't been on skis more than 18 or 20 times in my life. It has stretched out over a good number of years, but so few times each year. But you should see the black and blue marks from the other less successful times!

Again time runs short and I have just barely touched on what I have been doing. Oh well, these letters will act as *aides mémoires* when I get home and we can gather nightly around the fire while I elaborate and enlarge on these skimpy pages.

[I'm not sure we ever did reread them together and I wish I hadn't waited so long to reread them myself as in spite of their length and the often detailed accounts of people, places and events, too much has slipped through the holes of my memory. I sometimes feel I am reading about a stranger, not me. . . . goodness, did I really do that?!!]

24 March 1945

Dear Mother and Father:

What heavenly weather we are having this month. Almost uninterrupted sunshine and spring balminess. It is just nine in the morning and I am sitting in the office with the window wide open behind me and the sun pouring in on my back. I have a vase on my desk with a dozen tiny daffodils in it that I bought the other day from a little boy on the street for ten cents. And pinned to my tweed suit is a bunch of violets that I bought in the market this morning for about seven cents. The daffodils, crocus, little hyacinths, primroses and snowdrops, as well as a few other things I don't recognize, give one a wide variety. And the trees are beginning to bud and down by the river the pussy willows have burst their silver gray fur into big fuzzy green caterpillars. And I have such spring fever that I can hardly sit in the office.

Did I ever tell you about the wonderful Swiss dish called *raclette*, which is merely cheese melted on a shovel or something and eaten quickly while still soft, with a boiled potato and a pickle. Doesn't sound good, but it tastes heavenly. I had never had it before, but made up for lost time and had it twice in the last ten days.

The big event of the week was the dinner party I gave last night. But I must start about three weeks ago when John, to whom I had loaned a pair of ski socks which I first washed and stretched so they would fit him, brought me a pair of lovely long cable-stitched socks and asked me if I was as good at washing socks and not stretching them as I was at washing them *and* stretching them. I said I thought I could manage and whose were the socks? He said they belonged to a very charming chap named Peter, but he refused to tell me his last name or introduce me, which was the price I asked for my labors. But being a big-hearted person and feeling that washing socks, particularly for someone named Peter, really was a part of my secretarial duties (certainly as much so as feeding paregoric to my colleagues last June), I did a superb job of washing the socks, not stretching them by the merest fraction of a millimeter. Then a week later, while the socks were still on John's table waiting to be returned to their owner, a very pleasant man came in looking for John. I asked his name and he said Peter, so I took a chance and asked him if the socks had been returned and were satisfactory. He looked a little startled and then admitted that was what he had come for. And thus started a lovely friendship. I met his wife that evening at a party and we amused everyone with the story of the socks. Jane (his wife) said that she was going to make up packages of socks and send them to me every week and please could I do the darning too!

Then they asked me for dinner the middle of the week, and so last night I asked them for dinner. I was a little scared, for dinner for four is quite different from dinner for two, and I didn't really know them terribly well. But, if I do say so, it was a terrific success.

Whoops, here comes the Boss.

30 March 1945

Dear Mother and Father:

This will probably be a most uninspired letter. The weather has been dreadful all week, I have had two new secretaries to break in (and they have more nearly broken me) and to top it all off, I have my first real cold *cum* sinusitis.

Much to my joy, last week I got a letter from the Andrés [with whom I had lived in Algiers]. Something had happened to the first page of the letter, but the rest was full of news of them and good wishes and affectionate regards to me. Those months with them are something that I will never forget. Hope that some day I will be able to go back and see them again. [Unfortunately I never did.]

In spite of hating the rain, it has done wonderful things to the spring and everything is four shades greener than a week ago. I hope to go to Zermatt for the last skiing next weekend and to Lugano the weekend after that.

Tell Richard to write. (Please)

5 April 1945

Dear Mother and Father:

This morning brought two letters from Mother and one from Father, all three most welcome. Glad that Richard is all right and that his leave is proving so pleasant. How nice that Joan can be there too—yes, I wish that I could make the four of you the five of us.

242

There isn't time to grouse in this letter about my so called promotion, I'll do that next week or maybe by next week things will be better. But they are pretty unbearable right now.

Amused at your comments about a roommate. The reason why some of Mother's words were underlined have become more apparent as the weeks have gone by and I am glad that my usual impetuousness didn't lead me into that mistake! However, I have been almost as impetuous and now do have a roommate. A nice girl who just arrived and who was pretty unhappy for various reasons, moved in with me last night. I think it should work out, at least for a while, as she is delightful and nice to have around. I was a bit surprised at my own dread of the actual moving in and have decided that the degree of my reluctance indicates that I really need a roommate for a while. There is no point in getting too used to living alone and liking it. And now that I have my own office and therefore some privacy during the day, I can stand a little more gregariousness in my time off. And I did feel like such a pig with that nice apartment and room to spare and having it all myself. Apartments are so hard to find and hotel life is so dull. And it wouldn't be for very long anyway, I don't believe.

Easter turned out to be a lovely day; Livia (my new room-mate) and I went to church together and then wandered around in the sun for a while. In the afternoon we went to hear *Parsifal*, which I had never heard before. The perfor-mance of course did not compare with a Metropolitan one, but being completely new to me I found it very beautiful and moving. I had expected to be very restless during a five-hour session of Wagner, but the time seemed incredibly short.

You will be interested to know that I heard the other day that the hotel where I stayed when I last saw Richard is no longer taking guests. Glad I didn't stay longer! [The Mount Royal Hotel at Marble Arch had been hit by a V-2.]

Deadline is approaching. More next week.

Dear Mother and Father:

Whoops, what a week! I moved into my own office, as I told you, and assumed my new duties which theoretically come under the heading of executive secretary but in reality constitute sort of a Mr. Anthony, Dorothy Dix and "Information Please" setup [popular arbiters of knowledge in newspapers and radio]. Anything goes wrong, anybody wants anything, there are any complaints, and from the Boss on down the problem is dropped in my lap. Rather exhausting but on the whole not too bad and often amusing. I am glad that I did not grouse in my last letter because many of those troubles have ironed themselves out and I think that the four of us may end up by being quite a cooperative team.

I am slowly getting organized, setting up distribution boxes for the interoffice material, put a blackboard up on my door to take care of notices for general consumption, and issuing interoffice memos on procedures. [This doesn't sound at all like me!]. And trying not to make myself too unpopular by insisting on a strict deadline for pouch material. It could be a lot worse, and I am really very pleased at having my own office, small as it is. It is the bathroom, really, and the tub is curtained off in one corner! But there is a pretty rug on the floor, a window by my desk, daffodils on the desk—the general effect is rather attractive. [Very convenient too, as was the tub for my weekly baths.]

I finally got to Zurich last Friday night. We had something urgent to take to the consulate and I didn't have anything to do and wanted to have dinner with a friend of mine there, so I volunteered to go. I left about five and there was daylight for almost the entire trip. Some day perhaps I will get *blasé* and unexcited about trips, but I am still all of a dither about the places I go and the things I see. The countryside is getting more and more beautiful and I kept my nose flattened to the window trying to see everything. (I had taken Emily Hahn with me to read, but never got further than the first page. Since then I have read more and enjoying it very much). The grass is now quite green and poking up everywhere are snowdrops and daffodils and primroses. Fruit trees are just coming into blossom, leaves are almost completely unfurled, gardens are being planted, birds are singing ... What is the use? One simply cannot describe it. It is like spring everywhere else, only three times as thrilling and lovely.

I was lucky enough to make the trip with someone who knew the country and he pointed out to me the castle of the original Hapsburgs, just a bit of a ruin on top of a hill. He also told me where there were Roman ruins and planned bicycles itineraries for me for this summer.

My friend and I had an excellent dinner and stopped off at a night club for half an hour before I took the midnight train back. It was a hasty trip but my first time to Zurich and it was rather fun.

Life with my new roommate is working out very well indeed. She is a nice person and a thoughtful and considerate one. A bit of a chatterbox, but nicely so. Her attitude towards me is a little similar to Joan's and I have the same big sister feeling towards her. So I am glad that I offered her bed and board. It has made a big difference in her happiness and thus to her usefulness.

She and I and one of the boys from the office left Saturday noon and went to Zermatt for the weekend. Here again words fail me in trying to describe it. It was a rainy gray day in Berne but we hoped that it would be clear further south. We had picnic lunches put up by one of the restaurants here and amused all our fellow travelers by our enjoyment of the ham sandwiches, cheese and apples. If you get out a map, you can follow our tip, along the Aare valley to the Lake of Thuns, down the lake to Spiez and then a sharp turn up the valley to Frutigen and Kandersteg, through the Lotschberg tunnel and out into the brilliant sunshine of a late afternoon in spring in the Rhone valley. We got dizzy trying to see out both sides of the train at once, and we made ourselves hoarse exclaiming over views of snowcapped mountains, straight rows of poplars along the banks of the river, tiny chalets perched precariously on mountain sides, meadows gay with flowers, and waterfalls leaping down rocky slopes. We changed at Brig, doubled back on our tracks on a lower level for a while and then turned up the valley of the Visp.

Our traveling was slower here as we were on a sort of cog railroad and from time to time had to proceed at a snail's pace because of avalanches which had swept away parts of the track, or half a bridge, and temporary ones had to be built. I have heard avalanches but never seen one in action— they are terrifying even at rest, the tumbled dirty snow reaching almost hungrily for houses and trees that it has just missed. In places the river was lost beneath the snow. Pastures and vineyards came right down to the tracks on both sides, when the slope wasn't too steep, and according to my Baedeker (which I read aloud to Livia and Marty during most of the trip) at one point we ascended "through the grand gorge of the Kipfen above the Visp, which forms a series of falls amidst huge blocks of gneiss." I'm not sure what gneiss is, but the rocks were huge and very spectacular. St. Niklaus was one of the prettiest villages, although the book says it is so surrounded by mountains that for weeks in the winter the sun never reaches it. It has a curious church with an oriental globe on the spire.

We got to Zermatt about 6:30 and were met by a friend of Cordelia's whom she telephoned to tell we were coming. He is a charming person and couldn't have been more agreeable, having reserved rooms for us, helped us rent skis, got a guide-instructor for Livia who had never even touched a pair of skis before, and made all the arrangements about bag lunches and so forth. We stayed at one of the smaller hotels but Livia and I had a corner room with our own bathroom and plenty of hot water (I often think that is the only reason I go away weekends) and with a balcony from which one got that lovely view of the Matterhorn. We all had dinner together and then our "host" took us out to see the town and for a bit of dancing. Most of the large hotels are closed for the duration but we managed to find good music for a couple of hours, by which time (having had so little sleep the night before) I was asleep on my feet. My escort, our "host," flirted with me in a delightful European fashion and improperly kissed my hand when he said goodnight to me—and of course I still get a kick out of that sort of thing. [According to the rules of etiquette, it is only a married woman whose hand is kissed, but I didn't mind a bit.]

Our trip back was a little less hilarious, as the three of us were tired and sunburned (Livia has been peeling all week but I have just looked sort of like a sunset.) Marty almost missed the train in Brig—we rushed on with the baggage while he went to buy us a bottle of anything he could find that was liquid. We got to the train just as the guard was shutting the door. We frantically told him we were waiting for someone and he kept pushing us in saying *"Il vient d'arriver."* Marty finally came rushing up the steps clutching three bottles of beer and we yelled at him to hurry up. He just made it, to our relief.

We got home about nine, gingerly washed our sunburned faces and fell into bed. (Anti-climax: I had been asleep half an hour when the telephone rang and I had to go see the Boss. So I didn't get to bed until 1:30, in spite of all my good intentions.) Our whole weekend, tickets, hotel, meals, guide and everything came to less than 100 francs. One of my Swiss friends, the girl from Thun who went skiing with us one weekend, wants very much a record of "White Christmas" sung by Bing Crosby. Can you do anything about sending it to me?

Package just received with orange and lemon powder and banana flakes! What a fascinating idea. Many thanks. Also Father's letter of March 24th. I have about come the conclusion that there is a job for me here for some time yet. This, as you once prophesied, is one of the most satisfactory jobs I have had, and I am becoming more and more enamored of my surroundings. So I may not accept that cook-housekeeper job after all. [I had facetiously suggested coming home and keeping house for them in New Hampshire.] But we shall see what the next couple of months bring.

19 April 1945

Dear Mother and Father:

Finally I wangled a vacation of sorts, leaving Berne Saturday noon and not coming back until Tuesday night. It was all too short and in spite of rigorous curtailing of social activities, I came back almost more tired than when I went, but it did do me some good and I did have a wonderful time.

The trip down [to Lugano] was scenic albeit uneventful, the only noticeable occurrence being my first meal in a Swiss dining car, a really very edible one. The fruit trees are in full bloom now and the meadows around them filled with flowers. Some places it looked as though it had been snowing, with the trees covered with white and the grass underneath also sprinkled with white.

The brilliant Ticinese sunshine woke me in the morning about eight and while waiting for breakfast (I was pleased at how my Italian had improved) I sat in the sun on my balcony (with just my pajamas on) and started the letter to you and took a few pictures. The mist was still rising from the lake, the church bells were ringing from the little church up the valley and under the cypress trees and poplars along the road, already dusty and white a few late church-goers were hurrying along. There was a farm right across the road and two colts, born on Easter Sunday, were playing beside their staid dams. Their legs were still uncertain and their love of adventure more imagined than real. They would venture across the pasture away from their mothers, only to skitter back again when the rooster crowed unexpectedly or the top heavy bus laden with *gazogéne* [a gasoline-saving device that made a gas fuel by burning wood or charcoal] and too many passengers rattled down the road. The lilacs were in bloom and wisteria hung heavily from the walls, both filling the air with their fragrance (which was later overcome by the odor of frying onions from downstairs), and by leaning over the balcony I could see the rock garden below, bright with its flowers, and the big bush of what look like giant peonies. As I may have intimated before, it is lovely country.

Monday morning was completely taken up with the preparations for and the duration of the service for Mr. Roosevelt [who died on 12 April]. I haven't commented on his death before as there seems so little to say. Whatever one's political affiliations, there can be no doubt that his death is most unfortunate and untimely and that it may have serious effects on the war and the post-war period. It has come as a shock to the whole world, and I was amazed at the size of the crowd that came to the services.

The trip back was wearisome, but just as we came down to the Lake of Lucerne from the mountains, a tremendous Wagnerian storm with thunder and lightning broke over our heads, and we rushed down the mountainside amidst the rolling of thunder and the brilliant jagged flashes of the lightning. Quite a sight.

Even four days away brought spring closer to its peak and the lilac tree outside my window is now in bloom, the grass green and all of us have spring fever.

My allotted time has more than run out and at last my conscience is bothering me. So I shall bring this to an end.

26 April 1945

Dear Mother and Father:

The poor Boss had gout again, which means he won't be in this morning, which also means that *maybe* I will be uninterrupted long enough to get this letter written to you.

Our housewarming was a howling success, and I picked the adjective on purpose. We had about twenty guests and they ate us out of house and home. Our new couch covers came just ten minutes before the first guest, several people sent flowers and everything was very gay and pretty. I served my usual beverage [a rum concoction] which met with the usual approval. And then we had a big bowl of little radishes which were devoured with extraordinary rapidity and were the most popular of our canapés. The others were salted crackers, sardines on thin pieces of toast, and round sandwiches of *pâté de foie, mettwurst,* and tuna *pâté.* People ate and ate, we had the radio on, some danced. The windows were wide open because it was so warm, so after a bit the police came and said they were glad we were having such a good time but with the windows open everybody else could hear and they weren't enjoying it as much as we were. So we closed the windows!

I finally pushed everybody out about ten-thirty or eleven, having gotten Livia to take the first contingent somewhere to eat. I of course gave the impression that I was coming too, which of course I had no intention of doing. I got the last guest, a nice young American doctor, down to the front door, persuaded him that I really did not want to go out and was just breathing a sigh of relief that I could go back and quietly pick up the *débris,* when he asked over his shoulder as he was going out the door "And what *are* you going to do?" Thoughtlessly I answered casually that I was going to fry an egg and perhaps have a cup of coffee. He did a quick about-face, came quickly back through the door that I was just shutting, and said "You talked me into it."

So there I was stuck with a supper guest. But he was quite a nice one, we talked medicine and surgery and hospitals while I made a salad of a lettuce and sliced cucumbers and cold Birdseye peas, put the coffee on for him, poured myself a glass of milk, got out the cottage cheese I had made that morning from soured milk, toasted Rye Krisp, and fried two eggs. While we were eating, he asked me for a knife, which I slapped into his hand in a reasonable facsimile of the correct surgical technique when a surgeon asks a nurse for some instrument. But apparently it was not quite right, so we spent the next ten minutes doing it over and over again until I finally did it to his satisfaction. It was most amusing, all the time he kept up a running commentary on operations and what he might really be needing, what made a good surgical nurse, etc.

But in spite of the food and the conversation, I got sleepier and sleepier until even he noticed it and went home. I finished clearing up and fell into bed. And all the next day people kept calling and coming in to tell us what a wonderful party it was and how much they enjoyed it. Our second installment comes off tomorrow—I only hope it won't be anticlimactic.

Oh, I forgot to tell you about our new icebox, which came just in time, for the party. A bright red Coca-Cola one, with *"Buvez Coca-Cola"* in large white letters on the front! It is very gay and giddy and fits in well with our red and white table cloth in the kitchen and the blue and white curtains. It cost us about ten dollars and we have a large block of ice delivered about twice a week. The weather is getting so warm that something of the sort was essential, particularly in our casual existence when we may buy perishables for supper and not get home to eat them for two days. I'll send you a picture of it sometime.

Our personnel troubles got so intense last week that I got as far as writing my resignation—but I think the chief thorn in my flesh read it when she was looking for something on my desk for she has been as sweet and cooperative as can be ever since, so I shall hold the matter in abeyance. Wish I knew what I really wanted to do (aside from the impossible of getting married). It would make life so much easier.

2 May 1945

Dear Mother and Father:

I am afraid that I shall have to give up my Italian lessons, as the lunch-time quota of jobs such as tailor, grocer, dry cleaners etc. will be so much increased by my "patient." I am sorry, as I enjoy the language and would have liked to become more fluent in it. The biggest event of this past week is my "patient" mentioned above. Livia went skiing in Zermatt again and broke her leg! Cordelia was with her, and the boy Marty who went with us before. Livia had her ski teacher but apparently got ahead of him and was going too fast, caught the tip of her ski (my ski, I mean) in the fresh snow and fell, twisting her right leg, and breaking it halfway between the knee and the ankle. Oskar [the ski teacher] carried her on his back and skied with her down to the next station. It was apparently a most uncomfortable trip as her leg was hanging more or less loose and every time he made a turn, it wrenched the leg.

Cordelia telephoned me about one o'clock that Livia had hurt her leg and for me to meet the 8:30 train with an ambulance. From her description and knowing that Livia was likely to exaggerate things like that, I didn't think an ambulance was necessary, but I arranged for our American doctor to be there and I got a big car. The train was a little early and the doctor was a little late, so Dan (don't think I have mentioned him before, sort of like Perry Culver [an early beau of mine in Boston]) and I rushed to find the second-class coaches. Just as we passed the baggage car somebody hollered my name—I looked up and there was Marty leaning out the door of the baggage car. He had brought Livia down on a flat sled and they had traveled the whole way in the baggage car. Both looked pale and wan from the trip, Marty because he is pretty young and was worried about his responsibility, and Livia because it was a rough ride and the only thing she had had was a little morphine by mouth a few hours before, which didn't do much to stop the pain. We got her on a baggage truck and I amused her with whatever nonsense came into my head until Bob came (the American doctor who was at our housewarming).

We took her down to Dan's apartment to look at the leg before deciding whether she should go to a hospital or not. (I was sorry that Livia had to hurt herself, but you can imagine what a good time I got out of the whole affair, helping Bob, boiling needles, holding Livia's hand and so forth.) It was obvious that the leg was broken, so we got the doctor from the M.A.'s [military attaché's] office who made arrangements for the ambulance and for her admission to the hospital here in Bern.

I rode along with her, went with her when they took her X-rays, and then to the operating room where they set it and put it in a cast. Unfortunately, the break was worse than they first thought and the X-rays the next morning showed that it must be set again and a stronger cast put on. So after breaking the news to the Boss (who was most annoyed, but I "bullied" him into writing a nice card to her and got him to authorize me to send flowers to cheer her up), I went back to the hospital and spent most of the afternoon telling her silly stories so she wouldn't worry too much about having to have it set again. Again I went with her, this time playing a more active part as I was asked to tie the tourniquet on her arm when they gave her the hypo to put her to sleep and later I had to take her pulse! (These bits of description are for Joan's benefit, as I don't have time to write a separate letter to her about it). She was moved to a private room and I "specialed" her until 9:30. It was not an arduous job, as she didn't completely wake up at any time, but it was a bit tiring, particularly as I didn't get any supper and I had been up with her so late the night before. And then it was emotionally tiring too. It reminded me a little of the time when I took care of the little French girl in Constantine.

It is a really bad break and it will be about four months before the final cast is off, as it is a double fracture of the large bone and what they call a greenstick fracture of the small one. I have persuaded Bob to keep her in the hospital until she can walk around a bit, either with a walking iron or with crutches, for I have neither the time nor the energy to take complete care of her in the apartment, and there are really too many inconveniences there for a bed patient—

besides not enough gas [which was strictly rationed] for three meals a day. [This despite an ingenious Swiss device that held an electric iron upside-down so that a pan could be placed on it to start warming.] I expect within a week or ten days she can get around a bit and within two weeks she should be back at the office. At least I hope so—frankly the thought of a twenty-four-hour-a-day roommate does not appeal to me, nice as she is. I find that I am enjoying these bachelor days again. But she is delightful and even in her groggiest moments Monday night at the hospital she kept worrying about whether I had had any supper or whether there wasn't something I wanted to do or whether she wasn't being an awful nuisance to me. (I am a funny prickly person sometimes, and find too much consideration and thoughtfulness as hard to live with as too little.) Oh well, it is good for the character and the development of patience and so forth, and it probably won't be too bad.

3 May 1945

Being 28 isn't too bad after all. And the news was a pretty good birthday present. Next best to the Armistice—and the weather cleared up.

The news to which I referred was the surrender of the Germans in northern Italy. Rereading these letters now and comparing them with later accounts of what happened during those weeks of negotiations before the signing of the surrender, I marvel at how successfully I concealed my participation. Insignificant as that was in the overall picture, nevertheless as Allen Dulles's executive secretary and office manager, I was obviously *au courant* with some if not most of what was going on. My trips to Lugano, which I wrote about as holidays, were that in part, but their purpose was to have me inconspicuously available if needed. Roosevelt's death, Mussolini's execution and Hitler's suicide had caused unexpected delays and complications. But finally the documents for an armistice on the southern front were signed on 29 April in British General Sir Harold Alexander's headquarters, to go into effect on 2 May. A "pretty good birthday present" indeed, which was soon followed by the even better and more wonderful news of V-E Day on 8 May.

Apart from my letters, my only souvenir of those momentous days are a few faded photographs of some of my office colleagues on the terrace of the villa in Ascona and a tiny china dachshund. This was named Fritzel after the dachshund which British General Terence Airey purchased (as the ostensible reason for his trip into Switzerland) while he was waiting with American General Lyman Lemnitzer at Allen's house in Berne for the message that would take them all to Ascona to meet with SS General Karl Wolfe.

10 May 1945

Dear Mother and Father:

Not much time for a letter this week, but I don't ever want Thursdays to go by without some sort of communications from me. You can imagine how hectic things are here, what with everybody excited over V-E Day. I still haven't really realized it and found it impossible to enter into the celebrations. But then I always have been sort of a contrary person—I will probably suddenly get excited long after everyone else has quieted down.

V-E Day I celebrated in my own fashion. Tennis with Dan, then the morning at the office, then Dan and I cycled to Muri for lunch where we ate in a garden under some big shady trees. We were through in time to ride a little further out in the country, which is lush and green and the air was hot and sweet with the lilacs and grass in the sun. We went back to the apartment for something cool to drink and I changed to a new gray "linen" suit which I bought here, and my new white shoes. I did a little work in the afternoon, the Boss came back about six, there was a cocktail party down the street at seven, I went to the first two acts of *Tales of Hoffman* and then rushed home and changed into a dinner dress and went around to the Boss's house for champagne out on the terrace. Then we went to the Bellevue for a nightcap and then I went home, in spite of everyone's protests. Berne was more alive than on New Year's Eve, with people dancing in the streets, the church bells ringing and the tower of the Minster lit up like a wedding cake. It really was exciting and for a brief moment even I felt light-hearted. It is wonderful to know that the war is over here, even though the worst is yet to come. Or am I just being pessimistic?

I have finally made known to the Boss what my wishes are as to the future [namely to go home as soon as possible, via Italy]. A vacation at home this summer is included in the request. So far he has not said yea or nay, so I still have hopes. Keep your fingers crossed.

15 May 1945

Dear Mother and Father:

A theoretically quiet week with the Boss away on vacation (believe it or not), but I find that with him away my duties and responsibilities are heavier than ever. And to make it more difficult, he took Mildred with him just in case he felt like doing a little dictating. Livia is doing the best she can part-time and on crutches which means I have to do a lot of waiting on her, and the other gal flatly refused to come in during the Boss's absence! So I feel at times like three or four persons rolled into one. However, the Boss telephoned this morning and wanted to know when I was going to get away—I explained that I couldn't very well leave the office uncovered, and he issued an order that the other gal come in and take charge from tomorrow on. I modified it a bit, as I have too much that I don't want to leave for her, but I shall leave early Friday morning and have another long weekend in the Tessin [i.e. the Ticino Canton region]. Livia and Spencer go tomorrow, one of the other boys tomorrow night and Dan and I Friday morning. It should be lots of fun. We are staying at a sort of inn about 15 miles outside of Lugano, where it is nice and quiet and nothing to do but swim and bicycle and sleep. Sounds vaguely like heaven to me.

25 May 1945

Dear Mother and Father:

The Boss took a "vacation" last week, as I think I told you and I expected to use the time to good advantage, catching up on the things that I never seem to find time to do while he is around. Having been ordered by the Boss to come down for a long weekend, Dan and I left very early Friday morning. It was a beautiful day, just hot enough to make one feel summery, and we got to Lugano in time for lunch with Mr. Bell at the consulate. After lunch Mr. Bell asked us if we would like to make a trip with him later that afternoon—I unenthusiastically said we would, as I could see no graceful way out of it, and we arranged to meet about four. In the interim Dan and I did a lot of window shopping and very little, for a wonder, actual shopping. We met Mr. Bell as planned and discovered, to my almost unbearable excitement and pleasure, that part of the trip consisted of going across the Swiss-Italian border at Gandria, which is just outside of Lugano (see your map). He had some influential Swiss friend with him who arranged the thing for us and gates were unlocked and we went through the short "tunnel" that divides the two countries. We weren't more than five hundred yards into Italy, but it was just enough to be thrilling and to make it more fun, there were a bunch of G.I.s on the other side, billeted in the tunnel. We shook hands all around and talked six to a dozen for fifteen minutes or more, until our Swiss guide said we must go back. Childish of me, perhaps, but I did get a big kick out of it and finally by my enthusiasm inspired even phlegmatic Dan into some semblance of enjoyment.

The planned part of our trip consisted of a ride across the lake in the customs launch to the custom house on the border on the other side. There we were taken on a conducted tour of the really extremely interesting museum they have made there, with exhibits of things taken away from smugglers, captured arms and so forth. We each of us got a souvenir of a little knife with a curved blade like a scythe.

Saturday I took an early train to Bellinzona and wandered around the town for over an hour before picking up my bicycle and cycling down the long valley to Ascona where I had a lunch date with Mildred, who had gone with the Boss on his vacation in case he thought of some letters he should write. The ride was long and quite hot, but fortunately mostly downhill and I enjoyed it very much. The Ticinese are friendly people and wave at one or say *"Buon giorno"* as you pass.

I spent the afternoon sitting in the sun on the terrace of the Boss's house on the lake at Ascona.

28 May 1945

Dear Mother and Father:

Rumor hath it that now we can send letters out more than once a week, if the pouch is not too big. So I shall try with this one and then write again, if only briefly, on Thursday.

I was telling Russ [a friend of my father's] the other day that you had moved to the country, and he spoke again with pleasure of the delightful lunch he had with you both in New York, of what an attractive apartment you had, and what a good lunch it was. He remembered particularly the delicious thin Spanish almonds that Gregory had brought for Mother. He is a nice person and my estimation of him has gone up by leaps and bounds since I discovered that one of his favorite records is Marlene Dietrich's "Frankie and Johnny" and that he is a Dornford Yates "fan"! Did you know him well?

Livia has been down in the Tessin for the last week, doing some odds and ends of work in the Consulate and theoretically getting lots of sun and rest. She was supposed to come back last weekend and as changing trains would be something of an ordeal by herself, I arranged to go to Lucerne to meet her and help her change to the train for Berne. But at the last minute Valla decided he had more work for her, and as there was no real rush about her getting back here, he said he would keep her for a few more days. (I hoped it would be for a whole week; I am ashamed at the way I dread her return, not because of her because I am fond of her, but because I really do prefer living alone and because of the additional responsibility it will bring into my already full life. So I have been very pleased that her weekend in Lugano turned out to be more than two weeks.)

However, since I had my room reservation in Lucerne and since I had been there only for a few hours once before, I decided to go anyway. I had picked a small hotel on the right bank of the Reuss and in the old part of town, the Hotel Balances. My room overlooked the river which flowed swiftly and noisily right under my window, and when I was out on the balcony I could see the lake, the covered wooden bridge with its stone *Wasserturm*, and Mt. Pilatus. It was a lovely view and to add to its beauty, the moon was full last weekend.

Sunday was bright and clear and sunny and a friend of mine offered to take me sailing. He had rented a fairly large sailboat and had packed a lunch, we took bathing suits (or rather wore them) and spent five glorious hours sailing down to Hertenstein and back. The wind was light and variable but we were in no hurry and just loafed along, dragging a bottle of wine tied in a string bag behind us until lunch time. There was a men's choir singing along the quay as we left and for over an hour the voices came to us on the breeze. The twin spires of the cathedral, the towers of the city wall, and the irregular roof line of the old city made a delightful picture at the foot of the mountains, with Pilatus wrapped in a swirl of gray cloud most of the day. There were lovely whipped-cream clouds along the horizon, the distant mountains are still snowcapped, the wooded slopes along the lake alternated with fields and impossibly picturesque *chalets*, there were a dozen or more other sailboats out too, and all in all it was just one of those unbearably perfect days. I got quite a tan, lot of fresh air and relaxation and my companion was most congenial. Absolutely nothing wrong with it except that it had to end.

Lucerne is, to my mind, one of the most charming of the Swiss towns. It is supposed to be a big tourist place, but in spite of that reputation it has managed to retain a lot of the authentic picturesqueness (or am I just a sucker too?). The streets were winding and narrow and cobblestoned, many of the walls of the houses are gaily painted with designs or flowers or real pictures, the fountains are all planted with geraniums. I fell completely under its charm and am glad that Livia's return next weekend will give me an excuse to go back.

4 June 1945

Dear Mother and Father:

Eleanor is using my typewriter and, as I had half an hour without too much to do, I thought that I would get out my Baby Hermes and write a note for tonight's pouch. Particularly as I have good news for you. At long last I have cornered the Boss and others concerned and got their agreement and approval to my departure from here on or about the first of August!!! So fatten up the calf and get out the band to welcome me home about the first of September, if not before! I really think it is safe to plan on it, as I can see nothing that could drastically change my plans. I have not yet decided just how or via what countries I will travel. By way of Alex Kirk [i.e. Rome, where he was the ambassador] if possible. I think that would be a lot of fun.

It was rather silly of me to write that news first, because now you will probably pay little attention to the rest of the letter. But do the best you can, will you?

Have you ever noticed that the most enticing country roads, the coolest and deepest woods, the hilltops that promise the most wonderful view, the most delightful little towns are always seen from a train window? And when one gets off the train or tries to find the same places with a car so that one may seek the fulfillment of their promises, they can never be found again. Very frustrating.

I was thoroughly annoyed by a dinner guest the other night who professed himself impressed by my efficiency and said that after the war perhaps my career lay in managing something like Bergdorf Goodman! I was furious. Think I shall have to dye my hair blond and get baby-blue eyes, so that people will realize that I really am not the managing type. I would so much rather be a clinging vine!

My half hour is up and Eleanor is through with my type-writer, so I shall bring this to an end. Not much point to it anyway, except for the news. Which I hope will please you. I am a little frightened at the idea of coming home after so long. Haven't any idea what I shall do when my leave is up.

7 June 1945

Dear Mother and Father:

Things have quieted down a little since the Boss is away and all our VIPs have left town. But I am still very busy and have time only for a short note.

One of the VIPs was my old friend Henry of the Frank and Henry Corporation [in Algiers]. He greeted me with open arms and for the five days or so that he was here I spent all my time following him around and taking care of him. He thinks nothing of calling one up at eleven in the evening to meet him to talk things over, or of having one meet him at breakfast, as I did one morning, to take notes on a conference he was having with the New Boss. (I got a good breakfast out of it too). It really is fun to work that closely with a person and to be given a great deal of responsibility and allowed to handle things myself, but it is exhausting too and I breathed a deep sigh of relief when he [the new boss] left. I think he will probably telephone you before you get this letter, at least he said that he would. He has asked me to stay here until his return, which should fit in perfectly well with my plans. But I told him that I would not wait if he was too long delayed.

I managed to get yesterday afternoon off, as Eleanor was here to take charge. (She is an extremely efficient and pleasant person, as I knew she would be when I was agitating for her transfer here.) I went down to Geneva for an afternoon of wandering and picture taking (pictures in my next). It is a delightful city but I still infinitely prefer Berne.

One reason I had been willing to make fairly definite plans to go home was that Allen Dulles was being reassigned to Germany and I knew, as I had said in an earlier letter, that working for someone else would be extremely difficult. Though sometimes irritating, he was charming and very intelligent, and I would have found it very hard to accept anyone new—in part because I felt he really didn't want to leave.

12 June 1945

Dear Mother and Father:

I had hoped that I would have time to get a letter out to you in the pouch last night, but I was suffering from post-weekend inertia and just couldn't seem to get anything done, except make plans for next weekend. Between one thing and another, I seem to merely exist from Monday to Saturday afternoon, the real high spot of the week being Sunday. I am beginning to dread my date of departure, as there will still be so many places I want to go to and so many things to do. Perhaps some day I will come back to Switzerland—but I am going on the assumption that I will not, and trying to crowd as much as possible into the next eight weeks. With the Boss away and the new regime not yet started and the unsettling influence of people leaving and arriving, my interest in my work has reached an all-time low. I don't dislike it, just don't care. And feel no compunction about arriving late on Monday morning and taking off an extra afternoon during the week. Well, I expect I have earned a little relaxation of that sort, moral and mental as well as physical.

Enfin and by devious routes I reach last weekend's trip. Get out your map of Switzerland and look for Spiez on the Lake of Thun about halfway between Thun and Interlaken. The train turns there and goes up the Kander Valley, the same route that we took when we went to Brig on the way to Zermatt. Just before the train goes into the tunnel under the Lotschen mountains there is a charming little village of Kandersteg. We got there late Saturday evening, in the midst of a misty fog which covered the tops of the surrounding mountains and made the mountain air even softer and more velvety than usual. And everything smelled so good, just the air itself and the pine trees and the pastures and faint elusive flower scents.

As usual I had relied on my trusty Baedeker to recommend a hotel but I had been too busy Saturday to make reservations. The Swiss have the hospitable custom of sending porters to meet every train, the name of the hotel printed in white conspicuous letters on their caps. I had picked the Victoria as being a good solid-sounding place but their porter was absent and the one from the Schweizerhof had such a nice smile that I let him take the bags. We walked down the village street, the mist soft and cool on our faces, the cowbells clanking as the herds moved barnward from the mountain pastures above us, unseen because of the low clouds.

The hotel was set in its own grounds, with its own little river, green-white and rapid beside it. The rooms were unbelievably comfortable and inexpensive and as usual the first thing I did was take a hot bath, with plenty of bath salts! There was a big Alpine Club Ball at the hotel that evening and the dining room had been converted into a dance hall, so we had dinner in one corner of the game room. The manager of the hotel, a very distinguished grayhaired chap, joined us for coffee and cognac in the so-called tea room, which was really an incongruously modern room with a bar, little tables around the wall, soft lights and a Jewish refugee who played the piano or alternately the accordion. A very pleasant atmosphere and our host was an interesting person to talk with. He was obviously the *pater familias* of the village and kept up a running commentary on the people around us: who was engaged to whom, who had had a baby, the jealousy between boys from different valleys. When a Swiss boy came to ask me to dance, he asked permission first of Herr Wirt and then of me. He told us of his duties as captain in the army and the troubles he had with the maids who were getting modern ideas and expecting to be allowed to dance with the boys from the village or the soldiers when they came in for coffee in the evening.

Herr Wirt [the manager] assured me that the weather would be good the next morning, but I felt it was just his optimistic nature. However, he was right and I woke to a bright and sunny morning, which was further brightened by what he called an "English Breakfast" of bacon and eggs supplementing the usual *café au lait*, rolls and jam.

The real point of going to Kandersteg is the walk up to the little mountain lake of Oeschinensee, which is supposed to be the most beautiful lake in Switzerland. It is just a pleasant distance from Kandersteg, taking about an hour and a half of leisurely strolling, uphill but not too steeply so. Many of the peaks were covered with clouds but the sky overhead was blue and the sun was out and the clouds drifted apart from time to time so that one caught glimpses of the snow-covered rocks on top of the Blumlisalp and the Frundenhorn. A brook ran brawling down beside the wide path, which first crossed a meadow as full of flowers as my most vivid imagination had pictured it and then through a little wood of evergreens. The ground was springy with moss and needles and the air, with its fragrance of pine needles and fresh-cut lumber and flowers, was almost intoxicating. There was still some snow, rather dirty patches I must admit, and there were dozens of waterfalls, some little ones and some where the water fell like a white curtain for hundreds of feet. I have never seen so many flowers and I picked a dozen or so which I have pressed and will send to you.

There is a little hotel right on the lake where one gets a very eatable lunch. It began to cloud up more after lunch and by the time I explored around a little bit and sat in the sun a bit and made a leisurely trip down, the sun was almost hidden and it had gotten much colder. The fresh air and sunshine had made me unbearably sleepy, so before my third bath of the weekend I took a nap. Again a pleasant dinner, coffee with Herr Wirt, a couple of turns around the dance floor with a Swiss boy and early to bed. Eggs for breakfast again, not too early (I told you I was taking Monday mornings not too seriously), and we were back in town again about eleven o'clock. And not in any mood to go back to the office. As I told you, I spent most of the afternoon planning where to go next weekend—I won't tell you now but wait until I have actually done it.

The amazing thing about this letter is not only that it is four pages long but that it is written two days before it goes out. Oh, I forgot Herr Wirt's comment when he came down to the railroad station to say goodbye, bringing me a bunch of Alpine roses: "But *no* Americans get to the station this early before the train!"

18 June 1945

No time for a real letter tonight—just got back from a lovely weekend and learn that I am going to Zurich to work in the consulate there for a few days. So I thought I would dash this off to you before I leave as I am sure I will have no time there. Should be fun, as well as a lot of work.

I accept with pleasure Father's offer of a job—making butter! Always did like that. Will the first of September be all right as a starting date?

June 19, 1945

Thought it would amuse you to get a letter with this heading [the Baur-au-Lac, a very posh hotel in Zurich where Father had stayed]. It won't be long or very inspired as Zurich is hot and muggy tonight and I am tired. Had to get up at six-thirty in order to get my "household" and affairs in order before I left. Valla met me at the train and he and Polly took me to lunch. After which I put in the hardest afternoon's work in a long time. Much less emotionally and nervously tiring than the three-ring circus I run in my own office, but five hours straight shorthand and typing is quite a strain on one's eyes and fingers especially when one is not used to it. But kind of fun, too, to cross off the pages of dictation and watch the neatly typed pages increase.

Now I'm back in my very pleasant and luxurious room at the Baur-au-Lac. One of the best hotels in all of Switzerland, I think. My room is facing the lake and I can hear the orchestra on the terrace below. I got into my housecoat, pushed the button for the waiter and ordered a lovely expensive meal—delicious curried chicken with rice, a large lettuce salad and a huge basket of black cherries which I shall nibble on all evening. Shortly I shall draw my bath, pour in handfuls of bath salts and go soak for a while. Lovely life of luxury, might just as well enjoy it while I can.

I'm enjoying Zurich very much. The office is the kind I like, small with everybody doing everything. Five men and me. I'm kept plenty busy, which I enjoy too. And Russ is a nice boss. Even takes me out to dinner sometimes! We had a wonderful dinner in the country the other night, a little inn reached through a covered bridge. We saw the innkeeper come in with the fish he had just caught—and ate them twenty minutes later with melted butter!

I'll try to get a long letter off, typewritten, during the week.

June 24, 1945

Dear Mother and Father:

What an incredible life I do lead! I'm sitting on the broad window sill of my room here at the Baur-au-Lac. (My four days T.D. [temporary duty] has turned into two weeks and possibly three!) The orchestra is playing softly on the terrace below, the fountain is splashing gently on the roof of the pavilion and the birds are talking sleepily to themselves in the big fir tree. The last bit of Alpenglow has just faded from the snowcapped mountains at the end of the lake and an incredibly large pale yellow moon is hanging over the lake.

And I was in Germany this afternoon! Just for about five minutes, as the Schnellzug [express train] from Schaffhausen rushed through the little bit of Germany between there and Zurich (see map), but it was long enough to be exciting and to enable me to say that at least I had been there. It looked disappointingly like the rest of the countryside, with perhaps fewer people, and if it had not been for the large Swiss flags where we crossed the boundaries, I never would have known.

Russ had to go on a long trip today, so I persuaded him to take me along in the car with him as far as Schaffhausen, so I could see the Falls of the Rhine. The day was hot and lovely, except for a brief uncooling thunder shower in the afternoon. I took the tram to Neuhausen and then walked along the bank of the Rhine, crossed on a bridge above the Falls, up to the castle and then down, practically into the roaring water it seemed, across below the Falls in a boat and then lunch on a balcony looking up at the leaping white river. A really lovely sight—hope my pictures come out. An hour or so of wandering around Schaffhausen and then back, through Germany.

I forgot to tell you that I saw a chamois on the side of the mountain the weekend I spent in Kandersteg! I was thrilled, except I had expected him to be white, instead of which he was a rather dirty brown.

5 July 1945

Sorry, but this will have to be short again. The Boss got back while I was still slaving at Zurich and "ordered" me back at once. So back I came, to have a delightful lunch with him, his wife and daughter [Joan] (a charming "child") before returning to work. He was in an excellent mood and Joan and I teased him unmercifully, to his apparent delight.

But he is off again tomorrow and we in the office are frantic trying to get everything done with and for him. So letter writing will have to be postponed, which is too bad as I am way behind in the accounts of my activities. But I hope to do better next week, when things have quieted down a little.

11 July 1945

Dear Mother and Father:

My correspondence has fallen off sadly, and I am most apologetic, but what with the Boss leaving and the new one arriving and all the confusion concomitant, and then all my own confusion about my departure and packing and so forth, there just hasn't been time to turn around, much less write long letters. Even this may be cut short, but I will do the best I can, and at least get last weekend's expedition down on paper. At least as much of it as can be confined by the restrictions of words and type and paper.

It is no use trying to make you guess what I did or where I went, because you would never be right in a hundred guesses. It all started because one of the people for whom I do some work speaks little or no French and somewhere he got the idea that mine was fluent. So when he had to make a short trip into the French zone [of occupied Germany] the other day, last Sunday to be exact, he asked me to go along to help him out with the various controls and patrols that one meets every five minutes. I jumped at the chance of course, and went up to Baden to spend the night, that being the most convenient place to where we were to cross the border. I was so excited that I could hardly sleep; I had been so afraid that I would leave here without getting across the border at all. It was a beautiful sunny day with big white clouds piled high on the horizon. We crossed the Rhine at Koblenz, and it seemed queer to go from a German-speaking frontier guard in Switzerland to a French-speaking frontier guard in Germany.

By the time we got near where we were going it was almost lunchtime, so we drove down a little lumbering [logging] road, beside a noisy brook, until we found an open place to have a picnic lunch. Imagine, picnicking in the Black Forest! I had to pinch myself to believe that it was true and had to keep repeating to myself that it really was the Black Forest—it looked so much like a New Hampshire woods and the brook sounded so much like a New Hampshire brook. The sun came slanting through the trees and white and yellow butterflies danced up and down the sunbeams. We sat on pine needles, the brook sang below us (of course we went wading in it after lunch) and I picked wild strawberries for dessert. There were even locusts to add to the familiar sounds, and the breeze whispered gently through the tops of the trees. I think my "boss" was a little amused at my excitement—I am sure he didn't realize just how thrilling it was to me.

After lunch we proceeded to do the business for which he had come—at one point during the drive we passed a slave labor camp, the horror of which did much to dampen my enthusiasm. It is queer how one thinks that one has complete realization of things read about, but when one actually sees a place like that, even though there are no longer people there in it, in a sudden flash you know that you haven't fully comprehended it at all, and there is a moment when you are terribly afraid that you may be sick to your stomach. I know that I am too emotional about things like that, and for that reason I am glad that I decided not to accompany the man I have been working for these last eight months on his next job.

It was still early when our business was finished, and I discovered that my "boss" had just "happened" to bring his fishing rod along. So we sought out a fishy-looking river beside the road on the way back, and proceeded to put the rod together. Then a most amusing thing happened. Along came a big French *camion*, passing us quite fast. A minute later there was a terrific screech of brakes and soon the *camion* reappeared, backing down the road to where we were parked. A couple of French officers got out and a very efficient youngster with a very efficient-looking gun approached us warily. They wanted to know what we were doing. My French came in very handy at this point and I explained we were going to try to catch a fish. They insisted on looking over the rod very carefully and in looking over the car very carefully. Convinced finally of our good intentions, they apologized and a little shamefacedly confessed that it had looked in passing as if we were setting up a radio, with the fishing rod as the antenna or whatever you call it. We all laughed and soon became good friends, they warned us about leaving the main roads, and told us some interesting things about the occupation and its problems.

They finally left and we spent about an hour fishing: that is, he fished and I watched and cut a stick to put the fish on and applauded each catch. (Only three little ones, but that was enough to be satisfactory) All in all, a very pleasant Sunday. And one that should make Richard green with envy.

18 July 1945

Dear Mother and Father:

Two difficulties to overcome in this letter, the pencil as well as my writing! Sorry, but I've been exiled to Zurich again, forgot my pen and have no typewriter available.

Exiled is perhaps the wrong word, as it is due largely to my own efforts that I am here, to do a bit of special writing. I find the change of administration even more difficult to cope with than I had expected and I thought discretion the better part of valor—discretion in this case being my absence. So I volunteered for this bit of work, after which I have permission to take three days off. Which will leave only ten more days to muddle through in Berne. Strange to think that this time next month I will be well on my way home.

Spent a quiet weekend in Neuchâtel last week. I was disappointed in the city but took a boat ride on the lake and got a bit of sunburn, which is most becoming.

Yesterday I took the morning off and rode the boat down to Rapperswal and back. Even more restful than usual as the talk around me was all Swiss German and I couldn't understand a word. I made the following disjointed notes in my notebook, which may help you get the atmosphere: poplars and willows with swans floating in their reflections; sunshine breeze and water with children's voices coming softly; a team of horses pulling a wagon and a young colt running alongside. Child teasing a swan; boy trimming a sailboat; splashing of a girl swimming; women with strong brown arms, washing clothes on the lakeshore. Mountains, clouds and church spire against the blue sky.

Will try to do better next week.

25 July 1945

Dear Mother and Father:

What with the heat and my excitement and packing and such, this won't be too coherent a letter. But as usual, I shall do the best I can.

Mail just arrived with one letter from Mother and two from Father—I am afraid that by leaving on Saturday, the last letter from Father to Berne will not reach me before my departure. I have sent instructions to Washington, Paris and London to forward any and all mail from now on to Chocorua.

Did I ever tell you about the window in the bookstore in Zurich which was filled with nothing but books by Hugh Lofting and by Beatrix Potter? I was entranced.

I got through my last tour of duty in Zurich in time last Thursday to get up onto the Rigi for the night, and spent

271

three days there. Wonderful views, nice walks, lots of sunshine. One of my pet barmaids from Berne was working up there for the summer and delighted to see me again. Her name is Lotti, a large blond cheerful person who knows something about everybody, I think. Tremendous amount of personality. The hotel is the old-fashioned pension type, with one's napkin safely saved in a little white paper envelope beside one's plate. Lots of children and old ladies and dogs. And I reminded myself of the people in Lisbon by taking fruit to my room after the meal. In fact, I spent a very salutary three days, being amused at myself.

I feel that now I can really speak French, as I have learned to interject a casual *"Tiens"* in my conversation from time to time. Been trying to do that for years.

Hope I can settle down when I get home, this traveling gets in one's blood. Decided at five o'clock that I wanted to go to Zurich for dinner last night, took a six o'clock train, had dinner and spent a pleasant evening and took the midnight back. Of course I am a bit sleepy today!

Things have changed here so much that I shan't be sorry to leave. The old days were fun, but it will be wonderful to be home again.

Have just reread many of your letters. Found it made me sufficiently homesick so that I can forget all the things I am leaving here that have made me happy. But as I said a few paragraphs above, it is all so changed that I don't mind too much. Even the apartment is no longer mine, but that is largely my fault, because I have been away so much and have disassociated myself from it.

I am getting a tremendous thrill out of casually saying to friends, "Yes, I am planning to be in Rome on Monday night!" Seems incredible. And even more incredible that a week or so after that I shall be home. Makes even travel-hardened me a little breathless.

This is enough of incoherency for one letter. I shall leave a letter, at least a short note and some photographs, to be mailed Saturday. I plan to leave here before noon, spend the weekend at Gletsch so that I can see the Rhone glacier before I leave, go to Lugano Sunday night and to Milan Monday morning—and Rome by Monday night.

Wish I could take longer and perhaps go by train, but I imagine Italy is terribly hot in August, and after all, I cannot have things *exactly* as I want them, even though I seem to approach a reasonable facsimile thereof.

27 July 1945

Dear Mother and Father:

Off tomorrow—And am I excited! still seems incredible and impossible.

Wish some day I'd learn to travel light. And simply.

31 July 1945

Dear Mother and Father:

I'm writing this letter as much for the sake of the letter-head FIFTH ARMY OFFICERS HOTEL, MILAN, ITALY, as anything. Isn't it impressive? There is an amusing story attached to my being billeted here, which I will tell you when I get home.

The weekend at Gletsch was wonderful and the Rhone glacier most impressive. I do hope that my pictures come out. Sunday night I met Paul (a colleague of the Paul we knew last summer) on the train and we drank champagne from Girolo to Lugano! Which gave me the proper rosy glow for my last night in Switzerland. Monday we lunched royally in Chiasso, crossed the border and drove to Milan. At one point, there was a possibility that I might drive all the way to Rome, but the car we intended to use broke down or something. So now I'm working on getting proper Army travel orders to cover the orders I brought from Berne, so I can fly to Florence this afternoon. Then to Rome tomorrow. It's a tough life.

Thanks for the cable—it came after I left but Paul brought it to me.

It's incredibly hot down here in the Lombardy Plain, but after North Africa and Spain I find I don't mind it too much. And it is all such fun. Except I wept on Sunday night.

I cabled Mr. Kirk [the ambassador in Rome] that I was coming and hoped to see him, but had no answer. Do hope he is there.

[Later that day]

Dear Mother and Father:

Just a brief note from Florence. Hot and dirty but I love it. Have a room with bath and hot water! Walked my feet down to the knees trying to see everything in six hours. And had three dates! One nice Welsh RAF officer who had dinner with me and we talked Dornford Yates and "The Saint" [hero of mystery stories by Leslie Charteris] among other things. Other two were two slightly inebriated young Americans who bought me a gardenia and took me dancing.

Am off for my next stop in a few minutes.

2 August 1945

Dear Mother and Father:

Here [in Rome] at last! It really doesn't seem possible. And it is all that I thought it would be, and perhaps a little bit more. I am now trying to arrange it so that I can stay over the weekend, but I am not sure that it will be possible. It seems so silly to me to rush to some other place to wait days and days there for transportation when I could wait here just as easily, but the Army is that way and there seems little that I can do about it. . . . The food is just as bad as ever, at least by Swiss standards, but it is rather amusing. I find it impossible to eat the large GI breakfasts but otherwise get along all right. Have a nice room in the Atlantico Hotel, a bath whenever I want it. . . . Forgot to tell you that the Sgt. who picked me up at the airport in Milan and had lunch with me did it, he said, because I smelt so nice! . . . Saw the tower of Pisa from the plane as we flew over. . . . I called Albert Horn last night when I got in and have an appointment to see Alex this afternoon and a date to lunch with him tomorrow. I am looking forward to that very much. . . . I know that it will be impossible for me to really see very much of the city while I am here, but I am going to try to hit a few of the high spots and take a few pictures. It is really rather frustrating to be faced with some hundred pages in a guidebook and to know that one has at most three days in which to do it.

5 August 1945
[V-Mail from Caserta:]

Dear Mother and Father:

Another lap of my journey accomplished. I did not succeed in persuading the powers that be that I could wait in Rome as well as any other place, and as soon as they were able to get through on the telephone I was ordered south. Oh well, I was lucky enough to have two full days in Rome, and at least I had that. My Thursday afternoon chat with Alex Kirk was very pleasant—I was amused at how little he looked as I had pictured him. And he is charming, but one of the most disillusioned and cynical people I have ever met. I had the feeling that he was wearing a mask, and that it might be rather fun and certainly interesting to see what kind of a person he was beneath the mask.

Friday, through the kindness of the ambassador, I was supplied with a car and a Roman-born driver, to assist in my sightseeing. It was quite a tour, and I was exhausted by Friday night. I shall try to sort out my visits and impressions and pictures when I get home, with the help of my Baedeker. We went to St. Peter's and St. John's, to the old Roman city and the Colosseum, down the Appian Way and through the Catacombs. The tour was interrupted at lunchtime by my date for luncheon with Alex. I had thought from the way I was invited that it was going to be a small informal lunch, but fortunately I took no chances and put on my best Sunday silk dress. It was a very large, hat-and-gloves-on lunch with dozens of people. I was met at the door as I came in by a butler with the seating plan, so that I would know ahead of time where I sat. Alex shook hands with me when I came and when I left, and that was all I saw of him. But luckily I sat next to Albert Horn, whom I found very delightful. John Walker from the Mellon Art Gallery [that is, the National Gallery of Art in Washington, DC] was also there—he had come down from Florence with me the day before, and I offered to give him a ride back to the embassy after lunch. My car was late, so we went up in back of the palace and called on the Princess Barbarini, who is a good friend of Mr. Walker's. She has kept large apartments in the palace, with some really nice ceilings. After that we did a rushing trip through the Borghese Gallery, with Mr. Walker pointing out his favorites and old friends. He has promised to take me through his gallery when I get back, and to lunch me. An interesting person.

Yesterday I drove down with some other people, coming through the famous Cassino valley. We were in too much of a hurry to stop to take pictures, but I was appalled at the desolation and destruction there. I am comfortably billeted here and hope to get off in a couple of days.

Epilogue

———❖———

On August 6 the B-29 *Enola Gay* dropped an atomic bomb on Hiroshima, three days later another destroyed Nagasaki, and on August 14 President Truman announced the surrender of Japan, marking the end of World War II. August also marked the end of a whole era in my life as well as the end of my wartime job with OSS. According to my little blue diary for that year, I left Caserta by plane on August 8 for Miami via Casablanca and then on to Washington for debriefing.

October, again according to my little diary, found me back in Washington, studying Spanish for some reason, and apparently still working for OSS, or SSU-CIG (Strategic Services Unit-Central Intelligence Group) into which OSS was reorganized. Then, in spite of the Spanish language studies, I left in January for a six-month assignment in Paris. I'm not quite sure, so many years later, why I accepted this assignment. Possibly the thought of actually living in

Paris was irresistible, or possibly because I needed a job and nothing else was offered at that time.

Whatever the reason, it was, as I wrote my parents, not a good decision. Professionally speaking, the work was dull and uninteresting in contrast to my previous jobs. I disliked my boss intensely, and I made medical history by being hospitalized with my third and most severe case of measles. But in spite of all that I managed to enjoy myself personally, primarily by making a number of weekend trips: Chamonix, Biaritz, Heidelberg, Brussels, Quimper, Pau and Lourdes among them. And even back to Bern for my 29th birthday. And again I wrote long, descriptive and I hope amusing letters, which don't belong in this book but may result in another short one some day.

My disillusionment with my job resulted in my resignation from the "Firm," as some of us still called it, in the fall of 1946, and my decision to apply to the regular Foreign Service. After several months training in Washington, I was assigned to Ambassador Robert Murphy's staff in Berlin; my parents were already living there as my father was one of General Clay's financial advisors. An unexpected bonus was that I was able to live with them, first in bachelor officer quarters in Berlin and later in Frankfurt when my father and I were both reassigned, respectively to the Joint Export-Import Agency and the consulate. An even more unexpected bonus—and one of the larger influences on my life—was that before I left Berlin I met my future husband, Louis Wiesner. He courted me long distance, traveling down to Frankfurt any number of times. We met in Washington where we were both assigned the following year and were married in 1950.

Looking back over the more than half a century, I find it difficult to identify with that adventurous young woman who seemed to adjust with astonishing flexibility to such a wide variety of unusual experiences. Yet if the immature youth is truly parent to the mature adult, some of the 1997 me must have been present then, as well as over the intervening years as I became a Foreign Service wife and mother of four children and then one of the first women in the United States to be ordained to the Episcopal priesthood. I have just recently celebrated the 20th anniversary of my ordination in the Washington Cathedral as well as my eightieth birthday. . . . Where, I wonder, will the Hound of Heaven pursue me next?

Between the Lines
was designed by Susan Lehmann of Washington, D.C.
The principal type is Adobe Caslon, based on a face designed by
the English type-founder William Caslon in 1725 which became the
standard roman face in Britain for more than a century. The historical
notes that open each chapter appear in Gill Sans, a modern sans-serif
paradigm designed in 1928 by the British polymath Eric Gill.
The book was printed by Thomson-Shore of Dexter, Michigan.

ISBN 1-889274-04-6

52195>

9 781889 274041

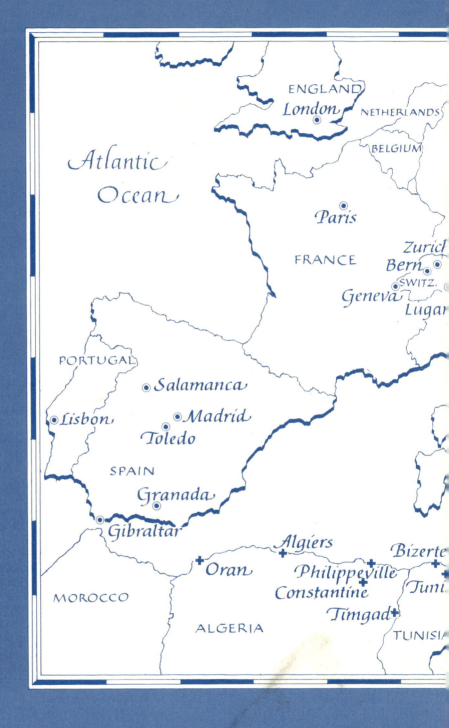